Welcome To Your MindBody

MIND YOUR BODY · MEND YOUR HEALTH

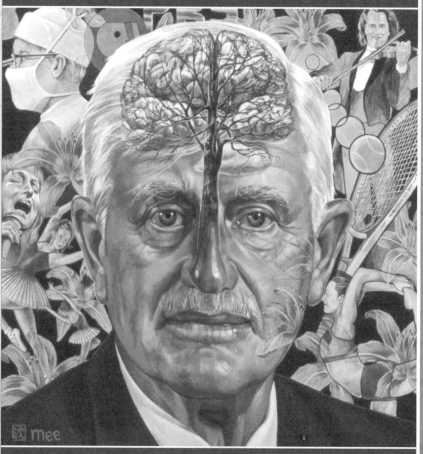

RUDY KACHMANN M.D. · KIM KACHMANN-GELTZ

Published by Rudy Kachmann, M.D. Behavioral Foundation, Inc.
www.KachmannMindBody.com

Library of Congress Control Number: 2007902825

ISBN-10: 1-933858-20-6
ISBN-13: 978-1-933858-20-3

Printed in the United States of America

For our parents, the greatest guides of zeal and persistence, passion and acceptance. And for our children—perhaps the most profound gifts from a parent to a child are love, faith and hope.

CONTENTS

AUTHORS' NOTE

The stories we tell are true. The names and certain details were changed to maintain confidentiality.

INTRODUCTION

I don't know how many times people have asked me what brain surgery is like, sometimes when they were only an hour away from finding out themselves. My job as a neurosurgeon involves the manual work of dissecting tumors, clipping aneurysms, and fixing discs, but my passion is the art of reconnecting the mind to the body.

The impetus for my interest in "mind-body" healing evolved while providing second opinions on surgical candidates who eventually confided in me that the cause of their debilitating back or neck pain was a deeply personal dilemma, stress at home or work, or a catastrophic loss in their lives, such as a divorce or death of a child, parent or friend. I often couldn't prevent them from seeking another opinion for a medical "solution" that in the end would offer only temporary relief. Suffering that emotional pain creates does not exist separate from the body.

As a practicing physician and neurosurgeon for 40 years, I've seen people beat the odds of death or disability, and others give up before the fight has begun because of a pre-existing depression. Sometimes there's a lot at stake—motor function, memory, vision, or even the life of a child. I am an unyielding believer in biomedicine's ability to overcome most of the challenges presented by a life-threatening injury or pathological process. But I also believe the abdication of treating the whole person, medicine's detachment from the mind, is a false, outdated dichotomy that scientific discoveries, contemporary needs, and economic realities no longer support.

Studies indicate that 60 percent of patients who visit doctors are suffering from symptoms related to psychosocial factors that cannot be diagnosed with standard medical diagnostics.[1] Medically unexplained symptoms spur about 5 percent of visits by children and adolescents to pediatricians and family physicians. Education is often more important than medication in these cases.

Medical circles still debate the notion that the mind influences health and illness. And patients may be confused by rapid developments in science and the outlandish claims for alternative treatments from none other than quacks. "Keep an open mind," I tell my patients, "but not so open that your brains fall out."

Scientific evidence links the functions of the mind with the health of the body beyond a reasonable doubt. Rapid-fire messages sent via nerve impulses but mainly slower-traveling "signaling molecules" keep the mind and body in constant communication. Tight communication allows each cell in the body to respond to the needs of the environment immediately.

Contrary to popular belief, the brain isn't an autocratic ruler. The brain is subject to signals from the cardiovascular, digestive, endocrine and immune systems. These systems in turn are subject to the brain. Many of the messages between the brain and the immune system stem from emotions related to stress. Contemporary life can unleash a flood of chemicals that are useful in the short term but toxic if they persist.

The biological mechanisms for disease and illness are rarely simple and straightforward. Yet standard medical care tends to separate the psychosocial components and treat the symptoms, a three-hundred year old legacy of the Enlightenment philosopher, René Descartes.

Mind and Matter

René Descartes believed that the "soul" was separate from the body but controlled our behavior like a ghost in a machine. To our ancestors, the phenomena of the mind seemed like a unique, special exception in nature, something attributable to unseen mystical forces. Descartes was a rationalist who believed that *thought* or rationalism was the only path to knowledge and proof of our existence. This became the first truth of his "dualist" mind-body philosophy, reflected by his famous statement: "I think, therefore I am." For Descartes and his followers, emotions were fleeting, making their relevance to health questionable.

Research by neuroscientist Antonio Damasio suggests that emotion is an essential part of the neural circuitry of decision-making and planning, and that the distinction made by Descartes between reason and emotion was an error.

Were it possible for Descartes to reappear at this hour, contemporary neuroscientists would also convince him that the mind is the genesis of neural circuitry and molecular biology. Technological and scientific developments of the latter part of the twentieth century revealed that the mind is made of trillions of tiny connections between neurons (brain cells) which reach into the body through nerve endings in blood, tissues, organs and bones. Nerve endings extend into the walls of veins and arteries, muscles, and the glands of the endocrine system to influence metabolism. Electrical impulses and chemical processes throughout the body (not just the brain) create different states of consciousness, including emotions. The state of the mind is merely a reflection of the state of the body.[2]

Cartesian philosophy led to scientific reductionism in medicine, the attempt to understand life by studying the smallest parts, then extrapolating from those pieces to form overarching theories about the whole. The narrow reductionist model provides a valuable intellectual framework to understand and evaluate disease on the basis of visible signs and symptoms but fails to consider the complexity of human beings. Our health and steadiness is a dynamic balance between mind, body and spirit.

Health care in the past was holistic, with enormous emphasis on the relationship between beliefs, emotions and health. Ancient Greek physicians used the term "holus" to convey how disease involved the whole person. With the discovery of germs and the advancement of sanitation in the nineteenth and twentieth centuries, doctors and patients began to lose sight of the connection between mind and body. The 1910 Flexner Report mandated that only medical schools that taught scientific medicine could produce certifiable physicians. A series of scientific breakthroughs had altered the values held by the public and the medical profession:

> Clinical and laboratory research had exposed the irrationality of "heroic" treatments (such as blistering, bleeding, and purging) and had proven the therapeutic efficacy and rational scientific basis of modern practices, such as antiseptic surgery, vaccination, and public sanitation. Most of the public and virtually all physicians now believed in the superiority of scientific medicine.[3]

As a result of Flexner's reforms, medical schools demanded anatomical knowledge and disease expertise. Today students study each part of the body separately, assigning organs and systems to separate disciplines such as neurology or cardiology. As a result, medical evaluations tend to be mechanistic and empirical versus empathetic, caring and educational. Many physicians today are no more than carpenters or mechanics of the human body.

With the aid of powerful molecular microscopes and advanced imaging techniques, scientists have gathered more information on the brain, mind and body connection than any other time in history. Mind-body science has verifiable proof, enough to make Descartes turn over in his grave. In Part I, we investigate the historical roots of the mind-body "disconnect" and how it continues to influence the model of American medicine and the view of the mind.

The Search for a Physical Link between Emotions and Health

In 1972, a pioneering neurobiologist and her team at the National Institutes for Health (NIH) introduced a revolutionary new method for studying the brain. Candace Pert, Ph.D., discovered the long sought-after opiate "receptor," the molecular key to understanding how powerful pain-relieving drugs like morphine can create the state of euphoria. Her research led to the discovery of a network of "informational substances" born at the cellular level and circulating throughout the body.

Thousands of different types of receptors sit on the surface of human cells. Receptors are molecules that sense, attract, and bind with specific types of "ligands," much smaller molecules. Ligand-receptor binding triggers a chain reaction of biochemical events involving genes and proteins. According to Pert, most of this activity takes place at a pre-conscious level; we only become aware of it when our emotional, physical or cognitive state changes.[4]

"Neuropeptides," the largest class of informational substances, circulate throughout the body and may be the biological equivalent of emotions. Receptors for neuropeptides are densely concentrated in the midbrain where many nerves converge called the periaqueductal gray or PAG, a key neural network that manages pleasure and pain. A dense concentration of receptors for neuropeptides also exists in the "limbic" region of the brain—a group of neural structures that encodes memories and regulates emotions. The limbic system integrates emotional states with stored memories of physical sensations, helping us recall things better. Anywhere the five senses enter the nervous system, dense concentrations of receptors for neuropeptides sit, ready for action.

Receptors for neuropeptides are also found in the body's network to fight disease, proving one of the most important physiological links between emotions and health. "Monocytes," immune cells that act to heal wounds and ingest foreign bodies, have receptors for neuropeptides called endorphins that lock onto the cells and influence their behavior.

Discovering receptors for neuropeptides throughout the body led to the view that informational substances, not electrical impulses, are the brain's chief mode of communication. But it's a two-way street: the brain receives direction from the body; the body receives direction from the brain. Pert used the metaphor of a musician to describe the effect of ligands and receptors on the body. Neuropeptides bind to receptors on neurons to adjust the body like a musician who modulates the tone of a musical instrument by varying its volume, timing and pitch. The "music" created is different states of mind.

New Notions of Mind

As we'll discuss in Part II, one of the greatest discoveries in science over the past decade is that the mind is more "plastic" than previously thought. Human beings are born with centuries of accumulated DNA which you can do little to change. But the complex neural circuits within the brain and nervous system that start taking shape before birth continue to grow and change throughout a lifetime. The brain only expresses an estimated 6,000 genes, out of a potential 30,000. Many personality traits are a mix between particular genes, environmental factors, and the brain's synaptic plasticity—the ability to change its structure and function in response to experience. Environmental factors trigger the constant give-and-take between genes and proteins within brain cells, reinforcing or pruning neural connections.

Neuroscientists have devoted a great deal of effort to investigating synaptic plasticity and how synapses adapt after a stroke to regain function. Normal brain cells are highly adaptable and can undergo changes in function and shape that allow them to take on the functions of nearby damaged cells. Healthy brains have tremendous ability to adapt and regenerate through learning and repetition.

Eric Kandel, Ph.D., a Nobel Prize-winning neuroscientist who set out to map the mechanisms of memory, believes that memory resides at the level of specific signaling molecules and their receptors. Memory is not just one big private library of the brain's hippocampus but rather, many different neural systems and subsystems.[5] With the aid of powerful molecular microscopes and advanced photographic techniques, neuroscientists can even see synapses change after repetition of a certain activity or routine. The brain is a malleable organ.

Today neuroscientists know a fair amount about how brain cells develop, how they speak to each other, what molecules are involved in learning and memory, and how they may be altered by disease or medication. They can distinguish numerous kinds of functions at work within the brain, each using different anatomical circuitry. With imaging scans, they can follow the traces of thought and emotion as it travels through various divisions of the brain. Until recently, it has been unclear as to what extent we can learn to control the activity of specific brain regions. Studies using hypnosis and biofeedback are proving that people can learn to consciously alter brain regions associated with the perception of pain.

No single pain center exists in the brain, but the rostral anterior cingulate cortex (rACC), a quarter-size patch in the middle-front of the brain, plays a critical role in the awareness of pain. Pain causes the brain to change. The longer you experience it, the more sensitized you become to pain and you can even become hyper-sensitized to it. Many chronic pain syndromes involve inappropriate levels of activation in the rACC that changes the way the region operates, a process called negative neuroplasticity.[6]

On the other hand, research suggests that practicing visualization and meditation changes the physical structure of the neocortex, the learning part of the brain that helps manage emotional stress. Meditation is similar to exercising, but the "muscle" is an area in the brain.

Richard Davidson, M.D., a renowned neuroscientist, compared the brains of Tibetan Buddhist monks with students of meditation over the past decade. During meditation, a Buddhist practice that focuses the mind on words such as "unconditional love" or "compassion," Davidson discovered intense activity in the monks' left prefrontal cortex, the region of the brain associated with positive emotions and idea generation. The brains of the students showed no such activity. The study supports the idea that mental training can increase the set point for happiness.

According to Davidson, we can think of things like happiness and compassion as skills that are no different from learning to play a musical instrument or learning golf or tennis. Like any skill, it takes practice and time to train our minds. On a deeper level, we can think of the daily practice of meditation or prayer as a spiritual path to a lasting transformation, a path to enlightenment.

The Unspoken Risk Factor

When it comes to self-care, most people already know about the health benefits of good nutrition and regular exercise. More often than not, doctors and patients dismiss the role that the mind plays in pain and illness. Negative emotions are the "unspoken" risk factor, in part due to the perils of misdiagnosis, pejorative overtones and medical bias. When you think excessively negative thoughts, you experience negative emotions and physiological responses like the body's stress response. Think fear, feel fear.

More than 50 percent of adults in the United States report feeling high stress on a daily basis.[7] No one factor determines elusive illnesses such as irritable bowel syndrome (IBS), fibromyalgia or chronic fatigue, but increasing evidence points to psychosocial stress as a co-factor. Doctors are reluctant to treat unexplained symptoms with unconventional therapies. Fear of war, terrorism, hurricanes, flash fires, floods or tornadoes, school violence, disability, credit card debt and racial injustice are just a few things on the minds of Americans today. Stress has a broad definition: "Stress is the inability to cope with a perceived (real or imagined) threat to one's mental, physical, emotional, and spiritual well-being, which results in a series of physiological responses and adaptations."[8]

Stress leads to activation of the "fight or flight" response to adjust the immune, gastrointestinal, neuromuscular, and cardiovascular systems to meet the perceived threat. Chronic activation of the stress response takes a toll on your body. Powerful hormones such as cortisol remain in the blood stream long after the experience of stress occurs, raising inflammatory markers and increasing vulnerability to symptoms that are difficult to diagnose. Long-term stress changes the central nervous system and the structure of the brain itself.

Emotions can even exist before cognition and be independent of thinking. When the door bell rings at 4:00 in the morning, your body reacts with attention and adrenaline before the brain can produce the experience of fear. Emotional processing involves the autonomic nervous system (ANS)—the division of the nervous system which controls involuntary activity such as heart rate and digestion. The body's stress response triggers the dispatch of powerful hormones in the bloodstream that generate arousal and anxiety. This activity causes digestion to stop, glucose levels to rise, and the heart to pump more blood to the muscles.

A stressful event can persist in the imagination and awaken other images buried in the psyche, images bound to repressed memories. The brain and body carry the burden of repressed memories, things in the past that have never been confronted or worked through. The nameless dread of repressed memories can eat away at immune function, creating susceptibility to illness. Recovery requires both self-awareness (personal insight) and physical release. Human beings are enormously complex psycho-spiritual-socio-cultural organisms.

Research reveals vast differences in the way people deal with identical problems. From a biological standpoint, individual brains vary dramatically in the number of receptors for biochemicals that influence behavior and "rational" decisions. People are wired with certain personality traits that make them more or less susceptible to disease and illness.

In my line of work, there is an epidemic of chronic musculoskeletal pain. The root of such pain often is an enigma—it doesn't relate to any structural problem, such as a tear, inflammation or nerve damage. Rather, psychosocial factors and the way the brain and nervous system process pain are ubiquitously interrelated with such pain.

Today's scientists are thinking about how the mind manifests itself in various parts of the body and how to bring that process into consciousness when treating enigmatic pain. The evidence is strongest for negative personality traits such as neuroticism, anger and hostility but studies also support that an optimistic outlook that generates positive beliefs, thoughts and emotions can improve health outcomes.

Negative emotions increase oxygen demands by the heart and the adhesiveness of blood platelets, raising the risks for stroke and heart attack. For men and women who already have coronary artery disease, anger can lower the pumping function of the heart to a lethal degree.[9] Stress can provoke an asthma attack. Anger and hostility also trigger the production of blood proteins involved in inflammation, contributing to the advancement of atherosclerosis, or hardening of the arteries.[10]

New research also suggests that affirmative emotions like laughter can help with sadness that often follows a heart attack by raising endorphins and nitric oxide (a chemical that helps dilate blood vessels). Laughter also suppresses levels of epinephrine, the stress hormone that constricts blood vessel function.[11] Research further suggests that laughter elevates a disease-fighting protein, B-cells, the source of a disease-destroying antibody, and T-cells, which help cellular immune response. Norman Cousins watched hours and hours of Marx Brothers movies and made it a point to enjoy a hearty belly laugh several times a day while recovering from a life-threatening illness. Laughter, hope, faith, and love are powerful medications.

Emotions sustain us, and serve to perpetuate the existence of humanity. Feeling connected to others gives us a sense of purpose and deepens our sense of who we are and our place in the universe. Faith in God is good for us. People who forge meaningful relationships in a church, synagogue or other community groups are less likely to get sick.

Hostility, cynicism and anger—negative emotions that separate one person from another—elevate the body's level of stress hormones, raising the risk of an early death. Depressed men and women exhibit all of the cardinal features of inflammation, the body's response to infection or injury, including elevations in pro-inflammatory proteins. Depression raises the risk for insulin resistance or pre-diabetes and even sudden death from cardiac arrhythmias.[12] A poorly managed depression can also lead to unhealthy coping tactics, such as overeating, alcoholism and drug abuse. Addictions will eventually lead to frustration, inner conflict and physiological imbalances that can lead to serious or even life-threatening illnesses. In Part III, we'll present how the mind may affect some of the most common illnesses.

The Power of Expectations

With all the medical diagnostics, devices and information available to physicians, you might think that a misdiagnosis is rare, but doctors are wrong 20 percent of the time. For example, let's say that you see your doctor for persistent back pain and she orders a MRI scan. MRI uses a strong magnetic field and radiofrequency waves that create clear pictures of internal organs, bones and tissues. After the test, your doctor calls to say the scan reveals drying out of the disc or "degenerative disc disease," and prescribes steroids and narcotics to manage your pain. Yet it might not be the cause of your pain. Back pain can become so intractable that it becomes a persistent presence, a constant psychic companion. The root of the pain may be forgotten.

Disc degeneration is a normal part of aging, not a disease, and nearly everyone shows some signs of wear and tear on the spinal discs as they age. And disc degeneration rarely causes persistent, unrelenting back pain. About 40-50 percent of patients are symptom-free within one week and up to 90 percent of symptoms resolve without medical attention in 6-12 weeks.[13]

Discs are like shock absorbers between the bones of the spine. They help the back stay flexible while resisting forces in many different planes of motion. Each disc has a firm outer layer containing nerves. If a disc tears in this area, it can be quite painful. The inside of the disc contains a soft, jelly-like core. When we are born, the disc is about 80 percent water. As we age, the disc dries out and doesn't absorb shocks as well. Adults may feel back or neck pain that comes and goes from drying out of the disc. But the body re-stabilizes any injured segments of the back. Even a ruptured disc that causes the agonizing pain of sciatica usually resolves within six months. Degenerative disc disease is a common condition that can be managed with conservative means such as stretching, yoga or chiropractic care.

In my experience, the diagnosis of degenerative disc disease alone has a powerful "nocebo effect"—a negative psychological, behavioral and physical response to a generally benign condition. Patients may begin to focus on their pain, start to guard their back, and feel justified to abstain from activities or pursue aggressive medical treatments. They may *expect* to be increasingly debilitated. Doctors in turn may crystallize the disability in the patient's mind by administering nerve blocks or steroid injections or other expensive invasive procedures.

Offering hope to a patient and can have a direct effect on the mind and physical health, a phenomenon known as the "placebo effect." Placebo effects are words, rituals or therapies, including surgery and inert medications that relieve or distract the mind from symptoms, and promote positive expectations. The placebo effect is huge— anywhere between 35 and 75 percent of patients benefit from taking a dummy pill in studies of new drugs.[14] Placebos can alleviate mild to moderate symptoms in part due to the body's release of endorphins. Within the context of this book, placebo effects include the psycho-physiological effects of meditation, faith, laughter, and the influence of positive communication on the severity of symptoms.

Conversely, the nocebo effect can result in the brain's release of stress hormones and in my experience (that I'll share in Chapter 7), can even contribute to sudden death. Beliefs are powerful. The nocebo effect worsens physical symptoms. After researching deaths by voodoo, Harvard physiologist Walter Cannon concluded that humans could die from "the fatal power of the imagination working through unmitigated terror." Dwelling on worse-case scenarios can trigger the body's stress response, signaling the mind and body to act without a physical reason to do so. You are, in a sense, what you expect. Optimists tend to live longer than pessimists.

Pain is always subjective, and often enigmatic. It can have an undetectable or a non-physical cause, making it hard to diagnose and treat. Although pain is a physical sensation, perceptions of pain are influenced by genetic, social, cultural, and psychological factors, producing different sensations in different people. Psychological insight and self-care are central to the prevention and treatment of chronic pain. Understanding how to enhance the therapeutic benefits of placebo effect in clinical practice has the potential to significantly improve health care. Placebos are powerful indications of the mind-body connection.

Healing the Mind, Mending the Body

Physicians are beginning to reevaluate their understanding of disease and treatment as a result of the new science proving the mind-body connection. Conservative medical centers such as the Cleveland and Mayo Clinics now offer mind-body therapies alongside conventional medicine because rigorous studies support their use. For example, yoga has been found to ease low-back pain,[15] and acupuncture can keep away tension headaches.[16] Daily transcendental meditation, a technique that involves mental concentration and physical relaxation through the use of a mantra (a repeated phrase or syllable) improves blood pressure and insulin resistance in cardiovascular patients.[17] Exercise releases of the body's natural stress-busters, the endorphins. Mind-body medicine can improve immune system function. Progressive muscle relaxation, hypnosis, meditation, controlled breathing and visualization has helped in the treatment of some types of allergies, asthma, hypertension, migraine and tension headache, herpes lesions, irritable-bowel syndrome and fibromyalgia. Conscious breathing, such as Lamaze or the techniques taught in yoga are powerful. A wealth of data supports that the rate and depth of breathing produce changes in the quantity of endorphins released from the brain stem.

While a conventional physician might recommend dietary changes, exercise or even powerful drugs and surgery to treat a chronic illness, doctors rarely teach patients mind-body relaxation techniques. The current system isn't set up to reward providers and patients to pursue less costly but equally valuable avenues of health care. Mind-body medicine offers the chance to resolve the anxieties that define the psyche and cause chronic physical pain. The challenge—the art for physicians is how to recognize when non-drug, non-interventional therapies are appropriate.

Emotions, pain and memory are deeply intertwined. Our early and oldest memories are usually extremely emotion-laden. Do you remember the first time you touched a hot surface? Fear is a learned response. Images of the past can rule us. People who suffer traumatic experiences can develop overwhelming memories of unpleasant events; the "fight or flight" rush of adrenaline cements especially durable, almost obsessive memories. Highly stressful memories are stored in the brain's amygdala, and may not be accessible to the conscious mind. Memories of emotional experiences can influence the way we feel and act beyond our awareness, protecting us from danger but also causing unconscious stress. Mind-body practices can evoke a physical release that diminishes that psychic frustration and emotional tension.

Eastern healing practices such as Tai Chi have a profound way of connecting the mind with the body, offering a spiritual but non-religious outlook on well-being that can be tailored to suit your own belief-system. Mind-body therapies won't magically will away disease, but they can help prevent disease, promote healing and make coping with stress or chronic illness easier. They pursue a spiritual calm, emotional peace, and physical fitness, merging the holistic concepts of the lifestyles of the East with more aggressive medical concepts emerging from the West. Mind-body medicine offers patients combinations of the traditional and the holistic: diet, exercise, massage, and prayer stand alongside medication, surgery, and biomedicine's incredible machines. It blends high-tech health care with proven therapies to treat the whole person.

PART I
The Roots of the Mind-Body Disconnect

CHAPTER 1

A Neurosurgeon's View on the Health Crisis

If all the drugs of the day could be sunk to the bottom of the sea, it would be all the better for mankind—and all the worse for the fishes.

–Oliver Wendell Holmes

It doesn't take a brain surgeon to see that American medicine is a paradox. Extraordinary medications are available today to prevent and treat a range of horrendous diseases. Small pox has vanished. Vaccinations practically banished polio, saving millions of children and adults from disability, paralysis or death. Organ transplants—the first performed in 1952—are routine. Scientists are deciphering the genetic basis of many deadly diseases, offering the promise of a cure. Advanced emergency care is at your finger tips. Clearly, there's no better place to be than America if you're struck down by a serious illness or injury.

The paradox is that the US spends more per person on health care than any other country on the planet, but ranks *second to last* for standard health indicators such as low-birth weight, infant mortality and longevity in comparison to other leading industrial countries such as Japan, France and the United Kingdom.[18] The US performs three times as many invasive cardiac procedures, but has the highest death rate from cardiovascular disease in comparison to other developed countries. Americans also have higher rates of arthritis, diabetes, and high blood pressure than other developed countries.[19] We're not getting our money's worth for what we're spending. The crisis is in part due to American ideals.

Americans value the pursuit of happiness. And when something goes wrong with our health, we want quick fixes and the liberty to choose aggressive medical treatments. We're proud of our technology. At the same time, hospitals, pharmaceutical companies, device-makers and Health Maintenance Organizations (HMOs) want to maximize profits. As a result, prescriptions, testing and procedures are the standard metrics of care. Author Norman Cousins noted in his classic, *The Anatomy of an Illness*:

Most people seem to feel their complaints are not taken seriously unless they are in possession of a little slip of paper with indecipherable but magic markings. To the patient, a prescription is a certificate of assured recovery. It is the doctor's IOU that promise good health. It is the psychological umbilical cord that provides a nourishing and continuing connection between physician and patient.[20]

Prescription medications rose to dominance in the twentieth century due to the development of vaccines and antibiotics that treat infection. Today almost half of the US population takes at least one prescription medicine, and one in six Americans takes three or more medications.[21] Spending on all forms of drugs to treat childhood behavioral problems rose over 75 percent in the past decade. Prescription drugs are the fastest-growing part of health care spending.[22]

The drug industry bombards us with direct-to-consumer ads that promise everything from a cure for insomnia and erectile dysfunction to the eradication of toe-nail fungus and depression. "No face, mouth open ... that's how the drug companies see the public," said comedian Jerry Seinfeld. According to John Abramson, M.D., a clinical instructor at Harvard Medical School and author of *Overdosed America*, "the pharmaceutical industry is raking in unheard of profits—more than three times the average of the other Fortune 500 industries" with annual worldwide revenues of $400 billion.[23] Abramson's extensive research revealed that drugs marketed as "cutting-edge" show little or no benefit in comparison to older, less-expensive medications. "Findings that support drug sales tend to get published in medical journals, and become accepted as fact. Unfavorable findings often don't see the light of day."[24] In 2002, the *New England Journal of Medicine* (NEJM) declared that they were dropping the policy that authors who review medical studies couldn't have financial ties to drug companies because they could no longer find enough independent experts.

America medicine tends to be a discipline of urgency. We can't wait for a drug to be refined, as we would wait for a wine to age, as a disease ravages society or our minds and bodies. The FDA's expedited review process and the push by Big Pharma to get their wares out the door and into the hands of doctors raise serious safety questions. Medical device makers and pharmaceutical companies spend more money on gifts to health care providers than they do on research.

They support 90 percent of the cost of continuing medical education classes at some of the most exclusive five-star resorts on the planet. Doctors spend much of their time promoting new drugs and procedures and testing them on patients, especially in hospitals. Key health care providers recently published a plea for more stringent regulations on these companies to better protect patients.[25]

The 10 best-selling prescription drugs treat such health problems as asthma, high cholesterol, schizophrenia and heart disease, all serious medical problems. Neurosurgery and drugs—antibiotics, ACE inhibitors, and AZT for AIDS and HIV, and medical devices— electrical stimulators for neurological diseases and implantable defibrillators for heart failure can and do reduce mortality and suffering. But with all our faith in biotechnology, we tend to dismiss the complexity and fragility of human beings.

The *New York Times* reported that rates for the most common form of breast cancer dropped a dramatic 15 percent from 2002-2003. Why? Because millions of women abandoned hormone treatment for the symptoms of menopause after a large national study concluded that the hormones increased breast cancer risk.[26] Recent news reports that drug companies played down the dangerous side-effects of profitable drugs such as Vioxx and the popular schizophrenia drug, Zyprexa raise even more concerns about the reliability of our sanctified medical remedies. Blind faith is bad medicine.

Almost 10 percent of the increase in health care spending over the past decade is due to angioplasty and stenting, but contrary to popular belief, the procedures don't actually reduce the risk of heart attack or extend life span for most patients. The best way to manage heart disease is through cholesterol-lowering drugs, managing stress, diet and exercise, rather than by opening up clogged arteries. Obesity and acquired diabetes, known risk factors for cardiovascular disease, are indictments of American lifestyle choices, rather than our health care system.

According to studies published in the *Journal of the American Medical Association* (JAMA) an estimated 30 percent of US patients receive contraindicated care, and almost 100,000 patients die each year from medical errors.[27] Medicine is an enterprise of constantly changing knowledge, uncertain information, and fallible professionals—what surgeon and author Atul Gawande refers to as "complications" in his book of the same name. Too many people believe that more aggressive treatments offer a new lease on life, and too many doctors prescribe drugs and perform tests and procedures for the love of money.

Diversity is one of the striking characteristics of our country, and should be one of our major strengths as a nation, but in the area of health, it isn't. A wide gap exists between Americans who enjoy health and those who are most likely to live shorter lives, according to a 2006 Harvard study.[28] An African American baby born is two-and-a-half times more likely to die in the first year of life than a majority baby. Life expectancy ranges from 84.9 years for Asian Americans while Urban African Americans have a life expectancy of only 71.1 years. Middle Americans have a life expectancy 77.9 years. According to the researchers, the disparities are due to preventable risk factors—smoking, alcohol, obesity, high blood pressure, elevated cholesterol, diet and physical inactivity.

Americans tend to be sedentary and eat more than they think. Brian Wansink, Ph.D., a food expert and the author of *Mindless Eating*, found that we tend to eat 20 percent more or 20 percent less without really being aware of it. And that 20 percent can creep into your waistband before you know it. "Just 10 extra calories a day—one stick of Doublemint gum or three small Jelly Belly jelly beans—will make you a pound more portly one year from today." Visual cues that prompt mindless eating saturate our 65-inch-wide flat screen TVs, big-box supermarkets and sprawling indoor shopping malls. Bigger seems better. Obesity is an epidemic that costs our health care system more than $80 billion dollars a year.[29] Childhood obesity has become a medical crisis.

I recently walked into a cath lab, a surgical theater where cardiologists perform invasive cardiovascular tests and procedures, and saw something I'll never forget: an adolescent boy stepping onto a bariatric scale wearing an adult-size hospital gown. His parents—both obese—looked the other way as he quietly read his weight to the nurse: two hundred pounds. The sudden silence in the room was conspicuous. I went over to the family and with their permission, said a prayer with their son. Ben went on record for being one of the hospital's youngest patients with acquired diabetes and heart failure.

American taxpayers are subsidizing the obesity crisis that in turn inflates health care costs. Agricultural subsidies got their start during the Great Depression, but today they're a form of corporate welfare. I love Indiana farmers and fresh corn on the cob but big agriculture uses about $40 billion in subsidies to crow corn that produces cheap high-fructose corn syrup, a stealth sweetener in many children's food products. Nutritionists blame the syrup for contributing to the childhood obesity crisis. Parents, read your labels.

Diets high in sodium, fat and carbohydrates are known to exacerbate blood pressure and the strain on blood vessels, arteries and the heart, brain and kidneys. If we choose to eat the wrong kind of foods over many years, certain genes are activated to trigger insulin resistance, high blood pressure and ultimately, heart disease. Research clearly shows that exercise and losing weight reduces all components of metabolic syndrome: blood glucose and hypertension goes down, HDL goes up and inflammation levels drop. All around us lay clues connecting disease to beliefs, attitudes, emotions and cultural factors— we need only to recognize them.

Americans also tend to overrate the effects of genetics and underestimate the influence of their own choices on health. Genes are turned on and off by internal and external influences. If you have a genetic predisposition to a health condition, you may or may not develop the disease, or suffer only minor symptoms. Nature and nurture, your family tree and your life experiences influence your health. We live our lives based on what we believe about ourselves, our capabilities, and our limits. And those beliefs in turn determine five critical variables that influence your health more than genetics: how you cope, what you eat, how you move, who you spend time with, and what you think.

The Lost "Soul" of Medicine

The hallmark of American medicine has been technological progress. People typically define progress in quantitative terms— growth in state-of-the-art technology and the innovation of new drugs to treat or prevent disease and illness. With this view in mind, medicine holds the promise of accelerated treatment through the quick identification of disease-causing agents. Patients who endure life-threatening illness or trauma may agree that American medicine is extraordinary. But according to the biggest study on US health care quality in history, day-to-day performance falls flat.[30]

Patient visits are rushed because doctors need volumes of patients just to cover overhead or turn a profit. Administrative expenses alone make-up 30 percent of health care costs. As a consequence in caring for too many patients, doctors may fail to accurately diagnose conditions or explain treatments, resulting in misdiagnoses, lack of patient compliance and complications. Americans spend almost $30 billion out-of-pocket annually on non-standard health care, a testament to dissatisfaction with standard medical treatments.[31]

The demise of meaningful patient-doctor relationships and the shelter doctors seek in drugs and technology are symptoms of the lost "soul" of American medicine. In popular medical lingo, the time-honored "stethoscope" is now referred to the "guessoscope." As few as 20 percent of new doctors, and 40 percent of practicing primary-care doctors can discern the difference between a healthy or a sick heart by listening to the heartbeat with a stethoscope, according to recent studies published in the *Journal of the American Society of Echocardiography*.[32] To compensate for the lack of skill, physicians may order an echocardiogram, an ultrasound image of the heart that can cost up to $1,000.

The decline of the stethoscope—a classic symbol of medicine—is one of the most dramatic indications that medicine has lost the balance between human skill and technology. Stethoscopes require a trained ear to interpret subtle sounds that can signal a leaking valve, blocked intestine or congested lung. And nothing builds trust more between doctor and patient than the laying on of hands. Although physicians have sophisticated devices including hand-held computers to assist in their evaluations, technology and instruments must not be used as justification for spending less time with patients. Effective medical care requires active listening and the ability to interpret emotions.

MRI Doctors

The invention of MRI was a powerful medical advance because the test reveals tissues as well as bones, enhancing a doctor's ability to detect and diagnose many diseases, including cancer, cardiovascular and musculoskeletal disorders. But the love of money or fear of malpractice litigation may pressure some doctors to test and over-test or inadvertently make an illness out of the normal process of aging, as in the case of degenerative disc disease.

What I call "MRI Doctors" profit from clever entrepreneurial schemes related to imaging tests. The most creative MRI Doctors procure referral deals with on-site radiologists or imaging centers who charge a flat fee for scans. The doctor-entrepreneur in turn bills insurers at a higher rate, netting an extra $200 on average per test. "Kickback" deals like this are illegal when Medicare or Medicaid patients are involved.[33]

Economic growth in tests and imaging over the past five years has surpassed all other medical procedures and evaluations.[34] Strong profits from tests and procedures helps explain why medical specialists enjoy a faster rate of income growth than primary care physicians who rely far more on cognitive evaluation and patient management to generate revenue. Doctors may feel justified to prioritize what reimburses well because of lower reimbursement rates, waning autonomy and higher administrative and malpractice insurance expenses. Taxpayers end up bearing the brunt of the cost.

Americans spent approximately $100 billion on biomedical imaging services in 2005.[35] Without an employer or insurance company brokering a discount, patients will pay full retail price for a test while a patient with insurance coverage might pay a small co-pay and deductible. Insurance companies, health maintenance organizations (HMOs), and Medicare use "black box" price databases to better negotiate with hospitals for volume discounts. In their book, *Critical Condition: How Health Care in America Became Big Business–and Bad Medicine*, Pulitzer Prize-winning journalists Donald Bartlett and James Steele note that "studies show an uninsured person who is not backed by the muscle of a pool is billed three, four, five, sometimes as much as ten times more than an insurance company whose patient has the exact same treatment."[36] Transparency in the pricing system would be another way to make health care more equitable for consumers.

Medicine and the Marketplace

The Medical Professional Corporation Act became law almost the same year I began practicing neurosurgery—1963. The statute was the first to recognize that medical professionals could be organized as a corporation and enjoy fees for services. Before the law, doctors couldn't take advantage of tax breaks and other favorable perks incorporation provides. The law was an economic boon to doctors but over the past 40 years, market pressures, administrative costs due to managed care, and regulatory constraints radically changed the philosophy and landscape of health care. Medicine and the marketplace began to meld with the advent of Blue Cross, Blue Shield in the 1960s—the same decade that government started to become the largest single health care payer in the US.

Today "fee schedules" determine allowable medical charges. And the fee schedule is predicated on two things: what the government says they will allow, which is Medicare and Medicaid, and what the insurance companies will allow. As a result, doctors often feel pressure to look for shortcuts and sure profits, sometimes to the detriment of quality and time spent with patients. Effective communication can result in better control of chronic illness and lead to shorter and less frequent office visits. But Health Maintenance Organizations (HMOs) who offer pre-paid medical care demand that staff doctors see as many patients as possible during the day. Health care is in part a business, but the benefits must outweigh the risks.

And then there's the infamous problem of access. The key determinants of health include genetics and behavior, physical and social surroundings, positive interventions that affect people's health, and *access to quality health care*. Access to health care is a major barrier to successful health outcomes in the United States. The rate of Americans without health insurance has risen almost 25 percent since the late 1980's.

The Problem of Access

When Medicare and Medicaid became law in 1965, Americans thought health insurance would be available for everyone. Today 46 million people or about 16 percent of the US population lacks health insurance. Lack of insurance means less preventive care. Some diseases, including arthritis, diabetes, and hypothyroidism can be subclinical before surfacing as clinical diseases with recognizable signs or symptoms. In the case of subclinical disease, prevention is paramount. The uninsured tend to have higher mortality rates than insured individuals. If you're a low-income family who earns too much to get Medicaid and cannot afford health insurance, the more problems you'll have if you or your child gets sick. Unexpected medical bills are a common cause of bankruptcy and mortgage foreclosures. And changing jobs often means changing or losing health plans—a big reason why people stay in jobs they don't like.

Health care spending is soaring, rising to $2.2 trillion or about 16 percent of the gross domestic product (GDP). Growth continues to outpace inflation and growth in wages for the average worker. Over the past 20 years, we've experienced a massive shift of health insurance risk from the government as well as the corporate sector, onto the balance sheets of working Americans. If the trend continues, Americans will spend on average $11,000 per year on health care in less than a decade.

Meanwhile American companies are competing against foreign companies that don't have health care costs because they're covered by their governments. General Motors chairman and chief executive, G. Richard Wagoner, Jr. sees rising medical expenses as the greatest threat to American competitiveness. Employers assume about 75 percent of the bill for private health insurance in the US.

During World War II, the FDR administration imposed wage and price controls to regulate inflation. Employers began offering health benefits to compensate for the lower salaries, and the federal government agreed that health benefits could be tax free. Many company insurance plans take advantage of the tax law by including frivolous benefits, such as "concierge" services to promote a more attractive benefits package. Between private and public coverage, corporate employees are over-insured, paying just 14 cents on average out-of-pocket, so patients don't have to think twice before demanding expensive tests or procedures. But that's rapidly changing.

As America moved away from a manufacturing-based economy to a service economy, and globalization transformed employee work patterns, employers began slashing health care benefits when costs began hurting the bottom line. The trend continues. Employees' share of health insurance costs rose 58 percent for a family and 63 percent for a single person from 2001-2006.[37] An increasing reliance on part-time and contract workers who are not eligible for coverage means fewer workers have access to employer-sponsored health insurance. The retirement of 77 million "baby boomers" will only worsen the crisis when the federal government supports Medicare with payroll taxes from fewer workers per retiree.

A Lasting Prescription

Americans can reduce health care cost inflation, meet the needs of the majority of people seeking medical care, and improve the quality of medical care while not growing government or raising taxes by adopting what Harvard Medical School professor and mind-body pioneer, Herbert Benson, M.D. calls the "three-legged stool" of *self-care*, medications, and medical procedures. "In this model, doctors go beyond the anatomical to address the framework of personal beliefs and behaviors that influence health, and teach patients how to break poor habits and develop positive attitudes and healthy behaviors."[38] Inexpensive mind-body therapies can lower the drug doses needed to manage pain and illness and lead to better stress management and disease prevention. One of the basic tenets of mind-body medicine is that people are active participants in their own health care:

Mind-body medicine focuses on the interactions among the brain, mind, body, and behavior, and the powerful ways in which emotional, mental, social, spiritual, and behavioral factors can directly affect health. It regards as fundamental an approach that respects and enhances each person's capacity for self-knowledge and self-care, and it emphasizes techniques that are grounded in this approach.[39]

Key benefits of mind-body medicine include reducing stress and promoting a state of relaxation; supporting the body's natural ability to heal itself; reducing pain and dependence on addicting pain medications; disease prevention; reducing the rate of infections such as the common cold; lowering blood pressure and glucose levels; improving intestinal health; and lessening anxiety and depression.[40] Mind-body therapies target the autonomic nervous system, the part of the nervous system that regulates many involuntary body functions, such as heart rate, blood pressure and digestion.

The legitimization of mind-body science led to the creation of the National Center for Complementary and Alternative Medicine (CAM) within the NIH in 1999. The center explores how complementary therapies influence changes in the brain and elsewhere in the body, down to the level of cells, molecules, and genes.

Some of the key tools that CAM-funded researchers use to explore mind-body therapies include genomics, chemical mass spectrometry (MS), functional magnetic resonance imaging or fMRI, and PET or positron emission tomography. Real-time imaging allows researchers to detect changes in biochemicals, metabolism and blood flow in the brain or other organs during mind-body therapies. PET research on the placebo effect explores how psychosocial dynamics such as conditioning, beliefs and expectations evoke physiological responses that affect neurological, immune, endocrine, cardiovascular, gastrointestinal, or other organ systems to relieve disease symptoms. Researchers affiliated with CAM are also studying the safety of herbs and dietary supplements and their influence on certain chronic diseases and the aging process.[41]

The research of distinguished Harvard medical historian, Charles Rosenberg, Ph.D. suggests that the wisest course in improving the cost and effectiveness of American health care is to adopt a *wide* view of health and illness, including that the mind can influence illness. A review of Western medical history in the next chapter will reveal how philosophy, myths, religion and science have limited or advanced our understanding of the mind and how it influences health.

CHAPTER 2

The Breadth of Mind

The wonder of the human body is not only the wisdom of its physiology but also the breadth of its mind.
                                        –Sherwin B. Nuland, M.D.

If you've stroked the forehead of a sick child, you know the feeling of wanting to "will" healing through the palm of your hand. This modest, voluntary action motivated by powerful feelings of emotion involves trillions of electrochemical signals, including billions of nerve cell impulses, several different hormones and the creative work of microscopic messenger molecules. If your brain were somehow isolated under the electron microscope during this deliberate action, you would see these delicate substances vibrating with energy and life. Or better yet, if you were laying inside a real-time fMRI machine, we would see that many specific parts of your brain were performing a sequentially precise, complicated neural choreograph combining visual, somesthetic, somatomotor, and other tongue-twisting terms. To coordinate the seamless integration of such spontaneous acts of love requires that far-flung parts of your body be in constant communication with one another. "The wonder of the human body is not only the wisdom of its physiology but also the breadth of its mind," says physician-author, Sherwin B. Nuland.[42]

The mystery for neuroscience, the science of the brain and the central nervous system, is how the brain and body communicate with each other to perform ordinary to extraordinary actions involving perception, emotions, judgment and behavior. From a scientific perspective, physiologies that integrate and coordinate disparate areas of the body—the interdependent harmonies that make us human, aren't so easily quantified.

Long before we had powerful microscopes and imaging technology to peer inside the matter of the cranium, philosophers, rabbis, priests, and even poets and writers pursued the riddle of the mind through the language of powerful metaphors: the soul, self, mind, free will or heart. Ancient metaphors illuminate something transcendent and eternal about the human condition, expressing the longing for a spiritual connection to something larger: "You will find me," God says in Jeremiah 29:13, "when you seek me with all your heart." According to some rabbinical authorities, the heart is equivalent to the mind. Judeo-Christian scripture locates many of the functions of the mind in the heart. When God offered to give the Hebrew, King Solomon anything he wanted in the world, Solomon asked for a wise and discerning *heart*. Many ancient cultures, including the Chinese, Indian, Mesopotamians, Babylonians and Egyptians constructed metaphysical concepts like the immortal "soul" to explain the breadth of the mind and address universal questions of our existence, including life after death.

The mystical tradition behind traditional Chinese medicine taught that the mind and body belong to an indivisible continuum with the heart as the bridge between the two. Western philosophers regarded the mind as something immaterial. Enlightenment philosopher René Descartes described the mental activities of the self as "soul," separate from the physical body but processing our environment and controlling our behavior in what philosopher Gilbert Ryle criticized as "the fallacy of the ghost in the machine." In Tibetan Buddhism, the word, "soul" actually means person or individual. Buddhism rejects the mind's alienation from the physical body implicit in the Western concept of soul. The transcendent view of the mind originated both in the ancient Greek view of a non-material consciousness, and in the Judeo-Christian idea of God in Genesis as a being outside of the world who created the world out of nothingness: "Now the earth was formless and empty, darkness was over the surface of the deep..."

To our ancient ancestors, the phenomena of the mind seemed like a unique, special exception in nature, something attributable to unseen mystical forces. Biological functions such as digestion and reproduction were reducible to obvious physical locations in the body, but emotion, cognition, memory and perception—consciousness— was difficult to pinpoint and explain. Bodily processes and states could be inspected by observations or dissections but the life of the mind was private and elusive to the observer. Historically, various human body parts were suggested as the core processing center or "seat" of the mind—the heart, diaphragm, liver, gut and brain. The difficulty of explaining how the unseen emotional and mental activities of human beings relate to the physical body is known as the "mind-body problem" in Western philosophy.

Healing and the Mind in Ancient Greece

Western notions of the mind originated in Greek myths and philosophy that contemplate the nature of space, time, substance and knowledge. Alcmaeon (circa 450 BC), the philosopher-physician and king, popularized the theory that the brain perceives sensations and is responsible for thought and memory. Hippocrates (460-370 BC) and his contemporaries, who were credited with writing the classics, *On the Nature of Man and On the Sacred Disease* advanced Alcmaeon's ideas about the tremendous influence of the brain, including the connection between the brain, emotions and physical sensations: "The body inevitably shudders and contracts when it feels pain, and likewise when it is overwhelmed by joy. This is why the heart and the diaphragm are particularly sensitive. Yet neither of these parts has any share in consciousness; rather, it is the brain which is responsible for all these."[43]

The famous Hippocratic Oath affirmed that there is an art to medicine as well as a science, and that ethics, integrity and trust are virtues that outweigh profit. The first part of the Oath establishes ground rules for medical society, including the obligation to share knowledge with other physicians. The second part of the Oath sets forth strict moral principles, including the prohibition of physician-assisted suicide and abortion which required the deliberate destruction of life. The Oath even deals with personal medical morality, such as doctor-patient confidentiality and sexual restraint. Hippocrates is our medical totem—a mystical icon that has philosophically shaped generations of doctors.[44]

Hippocratic physicians were remarkably ahead of their time, teaching that human beings think, see, feel and experience the world, as well as temper emotions and form memories through the brain. "From the brain comes joys, delights, laughter and sports, and sorrows, grief, despondency and lamentations. And by this, in an especial manner, we acquire wisdom and knowledge and see and hear, and know what are foul and what are fair . . ."[45] Today scientists know that emotion is a strong component in memory formation, and that people who suffer traumatic experiences develop overwhelming memories of unpleasant events; the fight or flight rush of adrenaline helps cement especially sticky memories in the amygdala.

Although it would be several centuries before intracranial neurosurgery would be ushered into routine practice by the pioneering endocrinologist and neurosurgeon Harvey Cushing, Hippocrates was familiar with the clinical signs of head injuries, and even created algorithms or rules to determine which type of trauma required immediate surgical interventions. Hippocratic physicians also classified seizures, head contusions, skull fractures and depressions and documented the surgical details of drilling a hole into the skull to relieve brain swelling.

Hippocratic physicians laid the groundwork for the scientific method of observation and experimentation, and were the first to posit that disease had tangible versus supernatural causes. Secularized medicine was born. Early Greek medicine and culture had attributed sickness to the scorn of deities. Disease the result of demonic possession or punishment in Homer's *Iliad* and the *Odyssey*. Greek legends about Asclepius, the mythical god of medicine and healing, held that miraculous cures were derived from divinely-inspired dreams that occurred while sleeping in his temple. Animal sacrifices were also a part of the healing ritual, including sacred serpents, symbols of rebirth and fertility. A rod entwined with a single serpent may have served as a rudimentary hypodermic needle, inoculating patients with therapeutic doses of snake venom. The rod also represented healing authority. Attacked by a plague of snakes in the wilderness, Moses holds up a serpent made from bronze so that the Israelites might recover from the bites. Today the "Rod of Asclepius" represents the American Medical Association (AMA) and the healing tradition of Western physicians across the globe.

A fundamental principle of Hippocratic medicine was to maintain stability of the body's four natural "humors"—black bile, yellow bile, phlegm, and blood which coincided with the four seasons; four qualities of the environment (cold, hot, wet, and dry); and four universal elements of earth, fire, water and air. Emphasizing the humors gave the Greeks a "reductionist" bias, oversimplifying the human body into organized elements. Most contemporary doctors are rational reductionists who believe everything can be explained by breaking it into its component parts. By analyzing the individual elements, physicians can discover how the parts act together to produce larger phenomena. After almost 40 years in specialized medicine, I've become an expert on understanding how certain symptoms often come together in specific groupings, and how some conditions follow predictably after others. If you end up in the ER with a spinal cord injury requiring urgent, highly specialized surgery, you want swift decision-making and precision in treatment. The reductionist medical model has taught me to see illness primarily in terms of disease and injury, which in many ways drives the excellence of neurosurgery. But medicine has become more and more dependent on the objective ways of science and dismissive of the subjective aspects of managing physical disease and illness.

For the ancient Greeks, health was related to the humors within the body and the outside environment surrounding the patient, a philosophy that was first developed in Eastern healing traditions thousands of years before the Hippocratic physicians. Traditional Chinese and Ayurvedic healers investigated the specific humoral disturbance that caused symptoms, which were then categorized and recorded. The humoral balance could also affect mood and personality. Health was a state of equilibrium and balance; illness was the result of an internal imbalance, or external influences from the environment such as the change of weather.

A person with blood as the dominant humor was said to be *sanguine*, flushed with color from too much exposure to the elements. *Melancholy* arose from drinking too much wine of the earth. If someone's personality had too much fire, they were said to be *choleric*, ill-tempered. A *phlegmatic* personality implied that the patient was apathetic, blocked like the congested nasal passages. Seasons, weather or even too much food and drink could throw-off the balance of the body's humors. Blood was hot and moist; yellow bile was hot and dry; phlegm was cold and moist; and black bile was cold and dry. Fevers made the blood run hot like the summer. The Greek physicians used herbs, diet, exercise and rest to restore equilibrium. Today the word "humoral" refers to "humoral-mediated immunity," the immune process involving B cells that act against bacteria and viruses, antigens that upset the balance of the body's homeostasis. Hippocratic physicians (and the Western medical model that ensued) worked hard to clarify and codify the humoral system which would lead Plato to lament, "The great error of our day in the treatment of humans is that some physicians separate treatment of psyche from treatment of body." The early Greeks had used the word "holus" to describe how health involves the *whole* person—mind, body and spirit.

Plato (428-347 BC) taught that the "psyche"—the Greek word for "soul"—was subject to emotional states, capable of virtues such as justice and courage, and responsible for planning and practical thinking. For Plato, philosophy alone was the therapy for sickness of the soul. He distinguished three parts of the psyche: the mind; spirit; and desire; which he referred to the brain; heart and diaphragm; and gut, respectively. He saw philosophers as "physicians of the soul, asserting that "physicians should treat the whole person, both body and soul, adding that 'if the head and body are to be well, you must begin by curing the soul; that is the first thing.'"[46] Plato proposed that the soul was an invisible essence given before birth and present in all *living* things. In *Phaedo*, he also develops the idea of an afterlife where good souls would live in happiness and light, and wicked souls would be punished. Platonic philosophy would have a profound influence on Aristotle, as well as Christian and Enlightenment thinkers who advanced Western dualism, the ontological belief that mind and matter are two different substances.

Aristotle (384-322 BC), a student of Plato, taught that mind and body were form and matter, inseparable parts of the same substance. Aristotle was convinced that the heart was the physical seat of the soul, and that the brain had no significance other than as a kind of radiator to cool the blood. He advanced a psycho-physical theory of emotions, describing anger as a seething heat in the region of the heart and a desire for retaliation. Aristotle also taught that truth could only reveal itself in moments of quiet contemplation, so mastering emotions was a virtue: "Anyone can become angry—that is easy. But to be angry with the right person, to the right degree, at the right time, for the right purpose, and in the right way—that is not easy."[47] Aristotle taught that we acquire virtues by first having put them into action—we become just by the practice of just actions. We become self-controlled by exercising self-control and courageous by performing acts of courage. He also advocated the curative power of emotions. In his *Poetics*, he argued that Greek tragedies stimulate pity and fear in the audience, which can serve as a therapeutic release or catharsis of unhealthy emotions.

Aristotle's heart-centered theory of the mind became the dominant view in antiquity and the medieval era, even though Erasistratus, an influential Greek anatomist and physician in Alexandria, had theorized that the brain controlled perception and movement. The Stoics (circa 300 BC) adapted the Aristotelian view of the power of emotions and taught that individuals could shift the mind by consciously analyzing a situation before making an appropriate response. Today we associate a stoic face with a lack of animation, and a stoic personality as colorless. The original intent of the Stoics was not to repress emotionality, but rather, use emotion as a source of wisdom guided by reason, especially in times of adversity.

Roman philosopher, statesman and orator Marcus Tullius Cicero (106-43 BC) wrote in *Tusculan Disputations* that in addition to care and maintenance of the body in healing, the art of healing the soul was a necessary component of care. Cicero referred to many physical diseases as disorders of the passions or disease of the soul that could be treated with words of consolation depending on the type of distress. Such views were regarded with suspicion by many, Cicero claimed.[48] The Roman view of the mind is mainly based on the theology-biology of Galen who many historians compare to the venerated Hippocrates.

Hippocrates was the model for Galen's medical thought. He revived the logical reductionism of Hippocratic medicine through experimentation, animal dissections and the Humoral system of diagnostics. Galen maintained a more Stoic, dualistic sense of soul and body than Aristotle, holding the soul to be superior to the body. Galen also theorized that the brain was the body's central organ or "the seat of the soul" breaking with the Aristotelian tradition that tethered cognitive and emotional significance to the heart. Through dissection of Barbary Apes, which are anatomically similar to humans, Galen discovered the spinal cord and nervous system and challenged Hippocrates' conviction that all brain wounds were fatal, suggesting a surgical solution. Although he would not dissect humans, Galen served as a physician to gladiators, giving him a front seat to view the anatomy of the human body under the skin. He also experimented with live animals, as Jeanne Bendick notes in *Galen and the Gateway to Medicine*:

> One of his methods was to publicly dissect a living pig, cutting its nerve bundles one at a time. Eventually he would cut a laryngeal nerve (now also known as Galen's Nerve) and the pig would stop squealing. He also tied the ureters of living animals to show that urine comes from the kidneys, and severed spinal cords to demonstrate paralysis.[49]

One of Galen's enduring legacies was to prompt physicians to attribute anatomy and physiology to the design of a "Supreme Intellect" or divine craftsman, a spiritual view that allowed Muslims and Christians to accept his system of medicine in later centuries.[50] His works were translated into Arabic, fueling the development of systematic Islamic medicine that would flourish, and even surpass Western medicine during the medieval era.

Galen also promoted interest in the "non-naturals," such as the "passions" or emotional struggles of the soul. According to medical historian, Anne Harrington, "The doctrine of the non-naturals was incorporated in medieval medical books alongside the Humoral system; it was important for physicians to help patients keep their emotions in balance, for the sake of their bodies as well as their mental states."[51] Galen attempted to understand emotions as mental phenomena with connections to pathological disorders, sometimes with success and other times failing.

A well-known case in medical history cited by Stanley Jackson in his book, *Galen—On Mental Disorders*, involved a young woman. After eliminating any humoral explanations for her physical symptoms which included palpitations, Galen came to the conclusion that she was unwilling to confess a secret love interest. He also observed that "melancholy women" were more prone to cancer than "sanguine women," a dangerous opinion that would influence the cultural view of breast cancer for generations.[52] In fact, the first contemporary assessment of the role of health risks in cancer deaths worldwide made no mention of mood as a risk factor.[53] Galen believed that many of his patients were cured by good counsel and persuasion alone and considered the balance of emotions as important as the balance of the humors, a view that would influence Western and Islamic medicine during the medieval era.

At War with the Passions

During the period of European history between antiquity and the centuries leading up to the Italian Renaissance, dogma advanced by the Roman Catholic Church dominated politics, art and culture. Science became the handmaiden of theology. The classical paradigm that had begun to rely on empirical evidence to support knowledge began to crumble. Religious orthodoxy substituted for observation, inhibiting curiosity, free thinking and learning. Christianity taught that the mind or its logical constructs—the Mosaic laws—couldn't restrain the passions as Aristotle had taught. "For I do not what I want, I do what I hate," writes the Apostle Paul (circa AD 3-62).[54] In this view, the mind and body were in opposition to each other; human beings were "at war with the flesh." The body was a temple; illness (evil spirits) invaded and laid siege to the fortress.

Medieval medicine was multi-faceted, relying on the skills of different classes of practitioners, including university-trained physicians, monks, and folk healers, depending on the patient's socio-economic class. In general, disease and illness were thought to be caused by a dissention of faith, rather than by natural sources. As people started falling ill from the Black Death, many attributed the disease to the sin and corruptions of the non-Catholics within their community. Tension grew between Roman Catholicism and folk medicine as the Church began enforcing Christian penitence, pilgrimage and prayer rituals. Herbal remedies, spells and incantations, and prayers led by female healers were directed at pagan gods as petitions to cure sickness. Religious persecution and "witch hunts" led to the trial, torture and execution of thousands of female folk healers and midwives who were associated with the work of the devil. Folk and secular medicine finally began to give way to monastic medicine which combined both spiritual and empirical healing remedies.

The father of Western monasticism, Benedict of Nursia believed that the care of the sick must be "placed above and before every other duty, as if indeed Christ were being directly served by waiting on them."[55] St. Benedict founded the monastery of Monte Cassino in 529 AD, establishing his Rule, a code of conduct for monks that would influence religious life in Europe for hundreds of years. His followers, the "Benedictines" developed monastic hospitals based on Galenic medicine throughout the medieval era to care for religious pilgrims and the victims of the vast epidemics of bubonic plague, flu, smallpox, leprosy, and other diseases that swept through Europe. Christian values, especially the precept to "Love thy neighbor as thyself," were strong ideals in caring for the sick and dying.

Throughout the medieval era, the collective consciousness hovered around the Judeo-Christian tenet of an unquestioning faith, hindering nearly all fields of inquiry, but also providing an ethical framework for the practice of medicine. Stanley Jackson in his book, *The Care of the Psyche* notes that medieval physicians believed healing prospered when the healer-suffer relationship was characterized by empathy and compassion, and suffered when profit was the goal. Jackson quotes a medieval physician as an example: "The art of medicine is rooted in the heart ... If your heart is just, you will also be a true physician. No one requires greater love of the heart than the physician. For him the ultimate instance is man's distress."[56]

Moses Maimonides (1138-1204), the medieval rabbi, physician and philosopher tried to reconcile an unquestioning faith with reason. He taught that there can be no contradiction between the truths which God has revealed, and the findings of the human mind in science and philosophy. Thomas of Aquinas, (1225-1274), drew upon Maimonides' view, arguing that it was possible to reconcile Christian faith with reason by acknowledging that immaterial realities such as the soul, angels and God could only be known through divine revelation. Faith was not based on reason. Maimonides and Thomas also advanced a psycho-physical view of medicine based on Aristotelian and Galenic philosophy: "It is known . . . that passions of the psyche produce changes in the body that are great, evident and manifest to all. On this account . . . the movements of the psyche . . . should be kept in balance . . . and no other regimen should be given precedence."[57]

Thomas thought that psychological and physical realities were identical in substance; cognition and sensation were the same processes of a physical mind. Philosophers of the medieval era only had vague notions of brain function. But a formidable counterculture in Italy was rising that would take bold risks and revolutionize our understanding of the breadth of the mind, world and universe.

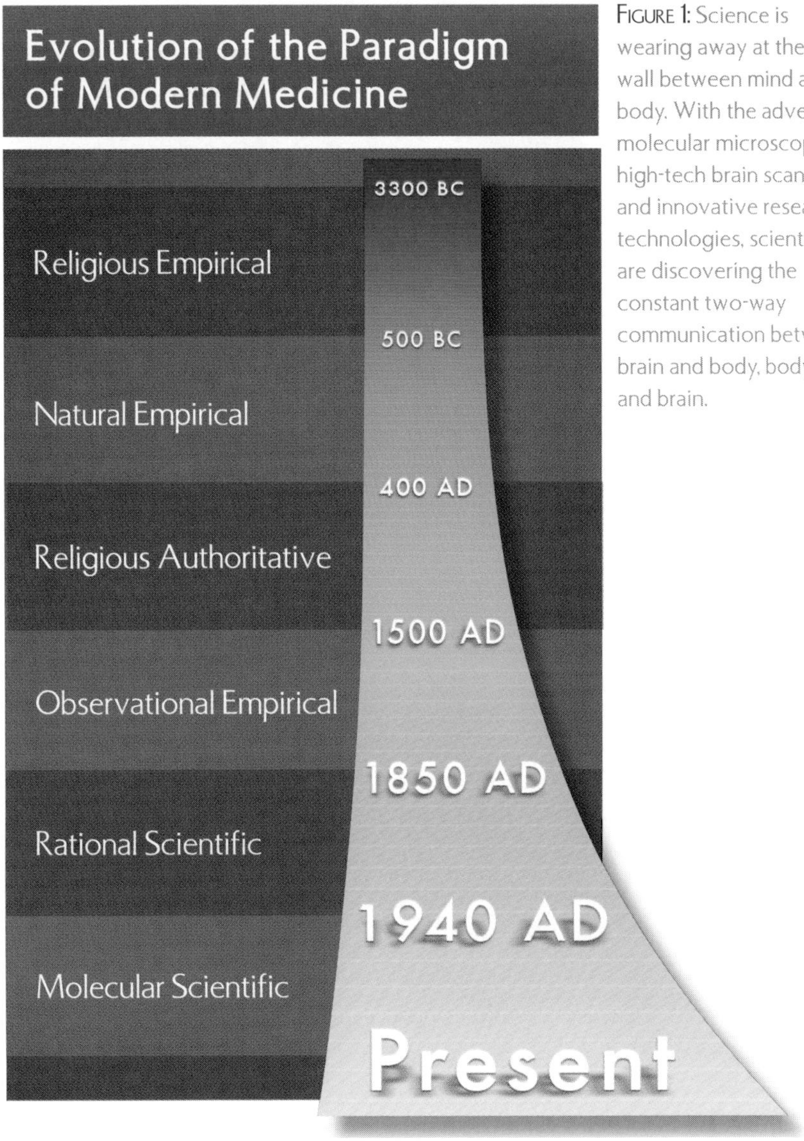

Evolution of the Paradigm of Modern Medicine

Religious Empirical

Natural Empirical

Religious Authoritative

Observational Empirical

Rational Scientific

Molecular Scientific

3300 BC

500 BC

400 AD

1500 AD

1850 AD

1940 AD

Present

FIGURE 1: Science is wearing away at the wall between mind and body. With the advent of molecular microscopes, high-tech brain scans and innovative research technologies, scientists are discovering the constant two-way communication between brain and body, body and brain.

CHAPTER 3

No Other Gods before Science

I think, therefore I am.

—*René Descartes*

During the sixteenth-century Renaissance of art, science, technology and culture and the era of the Reformation, the pendulum swung back towards the ancient Greek notion that illness was due to malfunctioning organs or systems—not malevolent spirits. The Renaissance was a revival of the best of ancient culture. Less than a century after Johannes Gutenberg's printing technology heralded a proliferation of books, Andreas Vesalius (1514-1564) broke with medieval tradition and authored the first anatomy textbook based on *human* dissections, seeking human cadavers from the grave and from the gallows. His *De Humanis Corporis Fabrica* contrasted Galen's description of assumed human anatomy with drawings of dissected human cadavers. Numerous discrepancies between Galen's text and Vesalius' diagrams were obvious. Vesalius bold dissections would earn him a death sentence, although his sentence was commuted. Author-physician, Esther Sternberg describes the risk involved in human anatomy lessons at the University of Padua in her book, *The Balance Within*:

> … legend tells that sentinels stood watch warn of the approach of the authorities. At the first sign of such an intrusion, the trapdoor underneath the slab was pulled open, allowing the body to slip away into the roiling river, now extinct, that then flowed directly under this hidden amphitheater. The professor was left innocently in his chair, lecturing alone to his attentive students.[58]

University education was typically under the authority of the Roman Catholic Church, but the Venetian Republic embraced intellectual and artistic freedom, exchange students and foreign enterprise to promote free trade and economic growth. As a result, students came from all over Europe to attend the famous University of Padua, including the Polish astronomer, Nicolaus Copernicus and English physicians, William Harvey and Thomas Willis. Harvey's *Essay on the Motion of the Heart and the Blood* (1628) mapped the human circulatory system and posited that the heart pumps the blood in continuous circulation. Thomas Willis published the first book on the brain and is blood vessels, *Cerebri Anatome* in 1664. Willis, the "father of neurology," suggested that different parts of the brain give rise to specific cognitive functions. He also pioneered the clinical and pathological analysis of diabetes, and was the first to identify "diabetes mellitus," theorizing that melancholy was the cause. In fact, it was widely believed that a happy state of mind protected people from all kinds of diseases and infectious illnesses, including the plague.[59]

Advances in technology, including the invention of the microscope, surgical techniques, the stethoscope and blood pressure cuff led to a separation of spiritual or emotional dimensions from the physical body. Vesalius' hands-on dissections and detailed anatomical diagrams allowed scientists to study human structural abnormalities for the first time, allowing empirical methodology to replace Galenic theories and guesswork. Author-physician, Sherwin B. Nuland notes, "In disagreeing with revered authority, Vesalius had demonstrated the importance of skepticism, of believing nothing valid unless it could be verified by anyone who took the pains to evaluate evidence."[60]

Medicine became increasingly specialized as researchers such as Harvey and Willis began to catalog human organs and systems and focus on their specific functions, leading to the Western medical maxim: "If you can't see it, it isn't real." As medicine further separated the mind and the body, physicians formulated concepts such as the imagination and emotional impulses that solidified the perception that diseases of the mind were "all in the head," and not based in physiology that could be seen. The French surgeon, Ambroise Paré even theorized that a woman's overactive imagination could affect an unborn child:

> Paré reported on two cases, one of a child born with the body of a calf, and another that occurred in 1517, of a child "born having the face of a frog," produced by the power of the mother's imagination. The mother, advised by her neighbor to hold a live frog in her hand as a means to cure her fever, was still holding the frog that evening, when she and her husband conceived a child.[61]

Paré was famous for saying, "Cure occasionally, relieve often, console always." Balancing strong emotions and restraining the imagination were important tenets of health during the centuries leading up to the modern era of medicine.

All Is Number

Artists have long looked to science for inspiration. Leonardo Da Vinci studied anatomy and engineering and applied his knowledge to the creation of lifelike visual art. Da Vinci's "Vitruvian Man" is the embodiment of Renaissance thinking, reflecting the emerging Enlightenment belief that humankind's perfection is dependent upon deductive reasoning, mathematical symbols and technical devices. In Dante the whole spirit of the Renaissance is to be found. Sir Isaac Newton's greatest claim to prominence came from his systematic application of algebra to geometry, and synthesizing a workable calculus which was applicable to scientific problems. "Man had been deceived by his eyes, his bodily senses—it was an instrument, Galileo's telescope and not the human eye that had revealed the true nature of the universe."[62] As Margaret Wertheim notes in *Pythagoras' Trousers*, thousands of years ago, the Greek philosopher, Pythagoras had created set of mathematical relationships that would describe the structure of the universe itself as "all is number."[63] The association of mathematics with a higher realm was easily imported into the Judeo-Christian context of Europe and primarily advanced by the influential Enlightenment philosopher, René Descartes (1596-1650).

Descartes reset the paradigm of modern science and medicine by dividing human experience into two distinct spheres: the mind, soul and the transcendent realm of God; and the body, matter and the mundane realm of the earth. What emerged from Cartesian thought was a determination to subdue irrationality, superstition, and tyranny and reduce everything to the logic of mathematics. Descartes helped advance the development of human autopsies by arguing with the Pope that the Church owned the mind, not the body. Separating the mind from the body meant that human remains were no longer holy or sacrosanct; the body was a corpse, becoming a scientific object to dissect, classify and study. According to Cartesian philosophy, the body can interact with the soul, but it was a machine, secondary to and separate from the soul:

> The crucial criterion for the existence of a human being is his or her ability to think, and this ability is completely independent from his or her body. Descartes goes so far as to say that he can imagine himself without his body. The body is of no use in proving the existence of a human being ... Descartes' world—including the human body—has a physical-mechanical constitution; it is a mathematical-geometrical construction.[64]

The Enlightenment marked a turning point for our Western understanding of the mind-body relationship. Reason was the path to reality, a point of view that still dominates our culture today. The self was discernable through intellectual intuition: "I think, therefore I am," said Descartes. "I concluded that I was a thing or substance whose whole essence or nature was only to think, and which, to exist has no need of space, nor any material thing or body."[65] The deductive and inductive reasoning implicit in contemporary science, medicine and psychology developed from Cartesian philosophy which introduced methodology for the systematic evaluation and verification if ideas. Cartesian rationalism became the most generally accepted attitude of the modern era, providing the building blocks for a renaissance of fast-paced, evidence-based increase in human knowledge, technology and power. Mechanization of textile machinery and other inventions such as the steam engine propelled industrial revolutions in Great Britain and America, improving cross-continental transportation and communication, allowing new ideas to spread quickly. Science became an abstract clockwork mechanism; the mind became the ghost in the machine.

Immanuel Kant criticized the assumptions of Descartes and earlier philosophers that man was capable of understanding "truths" through pure reason and thought. "Passions are cancers for pure practical reason and often incurable," said Kant in *Anthropologie* (1798).[66] Kant argued that the mind is an active agent in how we perceive and interact with the world; it creates reality just as much as it perceives it.[67]

Mathematician, John von Neumann was the first to show how quantum theory suggests a mathematical application for Kant's philosophy of mind. Physical objects would have no attributes if a conscious observer was not there watching them: "Consciousness creates reality." Contemporary neuroscientists Antonio and Hannah Damasio have built a strong case based on biochemical research that emotions are critical to human cognition and decision-making. Understanding and reasoning are not isolated or opposing faculties of mind; reason is imbued with emotion and memories.[68] "Descartes celebrated the separation of reason from emotion and severed reason from its biological function," said Damasio in *Descartes Error*.[69]

The freedom of expression in the art, music and literature of the Romantics was in part a protest against the emotional negation, order and logic, and spiritual alienation of the Enlightenment. "With all your science can you tell how it is, and whence it is that light comes into the soul?" asked Henry David Thoreau.[70] Romantic rhetoric advocated nature over artifice, country over city and heart over head. But anatomical studies and the new empirical approach to science and medicine advanced our understanding of the human body so remarkably that it became heresy to think of human beings in spiritual or emotional terms. Medicine began to look inward.

The cellular world exploded, increasing confidence in the marvels of modern medicine and further distancing the mind from the body. The founder of cellular pathology, Rudolf Virchow (1821-1902) theorized that the cell was the fundamental unit of life. Louis Pasteur (1822-1895) and Robert Koch (1843-1910) isolated disease-causing bacteria, demonstrating that microorganisms could cause illness. Physicians began to track and correlate specific diseases with treatment results, laying the groundwork for epidemiology.

After the twentieth-century discovery of powerful new drugs like antibiotics and steroids to treat infectious and inflammatory diseases, scientists focused on targeting the agent that triggers the illness and ignored the body's own natural defense against disease—the immune system. Disease began to have an objective existence, creating distance between the doctor and the patient, and the patient and the disease. Technology furthered the divide. French doctor Rene Laennec invented the stethoscope in 1816 to put some space between the physician and patient. Women didn't like it when doctors put their ears to their chests to listen to heart sounds. Curing an illness became a matter of science and economy, treatment standards that continue today.

The Darwinian Revolution

Another turning point in Western civilization took place in 1859 when Charles Darwin published *On the Origin of the Species*. The theory that human beings evolved from apes was alarming to nineteenth-century Europeans who saw themselves as the pinnacle of God's creation. Most people believed that the world was created in seven days as described in Genesis, the first book of the Bible. Darwin theorized that Homo sapiens came into being by chance in a ruthless struggle for survival. According to Darwin, the strong always overcame the weak, enabling advancement. Disease therefore was a natural phenomenon, not an experience with any moral, emotional or spiritual meaning. Modern science asks us to believe that living beings, in all their beauty and infinite variety, are the products of ever new combinations of nucleotide bases, the building blocks of DNA's genetic code. Darwin would influence the behaviorists who did not believe in a power beyond the material.

Darwin's ideas also challenged Judeo-Christian views on the purpose of science. From the time of Galen, science's ultimate purpose or end was to reveal the Creator's divine design of nature. For example, Sir Isaac Newton (1642-1727) said, "When I wrote my treatise about our [gravitational] system, I had an eye upon such principles as might work with considering men, for the belief of a deity; and nothing can rejoice me more than to find it useful for that purpose."[71] The bond between religious morals and science was broken by the Darwinian revolution.

Some argue that Darwinism became an instrument to verify the presumptive inferiority of women, blacks and Jews, and rationalize the politics of disenfranchisement and segregation into a social-scientific terminology. His second publication, *The Descent of Man, and Selection in Relation to Sex* had tremendous influence on ideas about the evolutionary roles of the sexes:

> It is generally admitted that with woman the powers of intuition, of rapid perception, and perhaps of imitation, are more strongly marked than in man; but some, at least, of these faculties are characteristic of the lower races, and therefore of a past and lower state of civilization.[72]

Darwin put woman on the evolutionary scale between a child and man, citing a study on comparative brain sizes to provide "scientific" proof that woman and "savages" were lower on the developmental ladder. "Man has ultimately become superior to woman," Darwin claimed.[73] A psychological campaign against women ensued that would be ludicrous were it not so lamentable.

Bigger isn't always better. Today we know that judging intelligence is much more complex than determining who has the larger brain: men and women have the same number of brain cells. Women even have more nerve cells in the prefrontal lobes than men, (18 percent). The prefrontal lobes are the "higher" functioning parts of the brain, regulating impulse control, judgment, language, memory, motor function, problem solving, sexual behavior, socialization and spontaneity. The prefrontal lobes assist in planning, coordinating, controlling and executing behavior. About 99 percent of male and female genetic coding is exactly the same but neuroscience and evolutionary psychology see some clear differences in that 1 percent. Psychiatrist Louann Brizendine notes in her book, *The Female Brain*:

> … scientists have documented an astonishing array of structural, chemical, genetic, hormonal, and functional brain differences between women and men. We've learned women have different brain sensitivities to stress and conflict. They use different brain areas and circuits to solve problems, process language, experience and store the same strong emotion.[74]

These brain differences aren't wholly immutable; social conditioning plays a large role in shaping gender roles. Paleontologist Stephen Jay Gould once said that "biology and environment are inextricably linked."

Evolutionary theory has been controversial throughout its history. Darwin's study, *The Expression of the Emotions in Man and Animals* offers an extraordinary perspective on the value of emotions within the context of biological evolution. Whatever your scientific, political or religious preference, evolutionary biology can provide a framework to elucidate many of nature's mysteries. And as with any scientific theory, research and time can strengthen or weaken that theory, or parts of that theory.

The current trend in "evolutionary psychology" attempts to explain certain mental and psychological traits—such as memory, perception, or language—as evolved adaptations. In explaining the epidemic of somatoform illnesses, for example, evolutionary psychologists teach that organisms are designed for particular environments. In other words, genetic evolution hasn't kept pace with social and environmental changes brought about by the advent of technology. We therefore often behave maladaptively in our current environments, much as a dessert coyote would behave maladaptively when transported into a rain forest. The immune system is a well-known example of a physiological evolutionary process. Antibodies are created at random and those that successfully bind to antigens replicate faster than those that don't.

Psychosomatic Illness

During the Victorian era of the nineteenth century, middle and upper class American women were expected to uphold and embody such cultural ideals as piety, purity, submissiveness and domesticity in the so-called "cult of true womanhood," a collection of attitudes that associated "true" womanhood with the home and family, (although by definition, women of color and poor white women were excluded).[75] A "true" woman was one who embraced her role as wife and mother in the domestic sphere, and refrained from activities outside that sphere, such as professional development or intellectual pursuits which were thought to overtax the female nervous system and cause symptoms of neurosis or "hysteria."

"Hysteria" comes from the Greek word for "uterus," a term coined by Hippocrates who thought the cause of hysteria was related to a wandering uterus that disrupted blood flow to the brain. Marriage and children (read sex) were the prescribed treatment for "womb disease." Hysteria was attributed to fainting, seizures, temporary paralysis, blindness, autism, abdominal cramps, vomiting during pregnancy, stuttering, numbness, aches and pains, uncontrollable laughter or crying, palpitations, trembling, headaches, lack of sexual interest ... and dozens of other vague symptoms that could not be verified with available diagnostics. In fact, after fever, hysteria was the second most common diagnosis in the seventeenth century and often became the catch-all for a variety of conditions in the nineteenth and twentieth century. According to a recent *New York Times* article, a 1965 study reported that "over half of the patients who received a diagnosis of [hysteria] would later be found to have a neurological disease; more recent studies put the rate of misdiagnosis between 4 percent and 10 percent."[76] Advancing technology such as the electroencephalogram (EEG) and computed tomography scan (CT scan) which can reveal brain lesions and other signs of pathology, would revolutionize neurology and psychiatry and eliminate conditions such as temporal lobe epilepsy from the under the umbrella of hysteria. The American Psychiatric Association finally dropped the term "hysteria" in 1952.

Hippocrates, Galen and several other medical authorities throughout the ages thought that "congestion" of the female genitalia was a contributing factor to hysteria; the 1899 edition of the *Merck Manual* even lists pelvic massage as a treatment. According to John Hopkins researcher and author, Rachel Maines, doctors and midwives would give women sexual pleasure to cure hysteria, first manually and then with the help of the vibrator after the dawn of electricity. "I'm sure the women felt much better afterwards, slept better, smiled more," said Maines. "The patient had to go to the doctor regularly. She didn't die. She was a cash cow." Sterilization and clitoridectomies also were not uncommon medical interventions, as doctors sought to remove what was thought to be the core of women's problems.[77]

Nineteenth-century physician, Paul Briquet finally laid to rest hysteria's historic association with physical disease of the female sexual organs. His decade-long, methodical observations noted in his *Treatise on Hysteria* (1859), found that married women were only slightly less prone to hysteria than unmarried women, and perhaps more importantly, that men could also develop the condition. Cardiopulmonary symptoms of "male hysteria" were recorded by military field physicians as "Soldier's Heart" after the French Revolution and American Civil War; and more recently "Shell Shock" or "Battle Fatigue" after World Wars I and II. Today the condition is known as Post-Traumatic Stress Disorder (PTSD), a psychiatric disorder that can occur after experiencing or witnessing of life-threatening events such as military combat, terrorism, natural disasters, automobile accidents, sexual abuse or violent crimes.

Physicians in the mid-eighteenth century, including Austin Flint began focusing on the nervous system as the locus for "functional neuroses" like hysteria in which no organic pathology could be found. The concept that physical health was somehow integrated within the mind or psyche evolved from the "Napoleon of Neuroses," Jean-Martin Charcot, who first identified, documented and defined the patterns of hysterical paralysis in 1860. Charcot used hypnosis to study the symptoms of hysteria, proving that the condition was not under voluntary control of the mind, and quieting scores of physicians and armchair critics who had believed that hysterical patients were faking it: "Is she hysterical or does she just hate housework?" Charcot believed hysteria was a neurophysiological phenomenon related to a hereditary weakness of the brain and nervous system that was possibly triggered by a traumatic event. Treatments for hysteria included hypnosis, electroshock, and the use of sedatives.

George Millar Beard, a prestigious nineteenth-century neurologist, redefined hysteria as "neurasthenia," a condition he associated with fatigue, headache, nerve pain, anxiety, impotence and depression. Beard theorized that neurasthenia was due to the unprecedented stress of the urban Industrial Age, including the inventions of steam power, newspapers and telegraph, and encouraged physicians to use the healing influence of the doctor-patient relationship to assist in recovery. His ideas were ridiculed and considered unscientific. Debate about what was organic illness and what was madness dominated the medical climate of the late nineteenth century.

Silas Weir Mitchell, a neurologist known for his studies on peripheral nerves, embraced Beard's theories on neurasthenia and prescribed bed rest as the treatment. Mitchell believed that intellectual, literary and artistic pursuits were destructive to the neurological and sexual health of "highly imaginative" patients, especially women of the educated leisure class: "Overuse, or even a very steady use of the brain is in many dangerous to health and to every probability of future womanly usefulness," said Mitchell.[78] Three of the best-known patients (or victims) of the "rest-cure" were Alice James, Marcel Proust and Charlotte Perkins Gilman.

Gilman experienced symptoms related to what is now known as postpartum depression, and wrote an indictment about her near-maddening experience with the "rest-cure" in her semi-autobiographical short fiction, "The Yellow Wallpaper" (1892). In the story, the main character retreats to a country house where she's kept in a room decorated with yellow wallpaper and not allowed to read, to write, or even see her newborn child. She gradually goes mad, pacing the room to trace the pattern of the wallpaper over and over again in an obsessive, endless plight to escape. Gilman sent the story to

Mitchell who privately admitted to friends that he withdrew the rest-cure as a treatment of choice.

With the advent of therapy developed by Sigmund Freud and Carl Jung, the rest-cure finally sank into obscurity as quackery but debate about psychological roots of hysteria continued. In *Studies in Hysteria* (1895), Freud theorized that hysteria may relate to something repressed in the psyche versus the nervous system. He believed everyone was vulnerable to hysterical illness, even himself:

> "I have never before even imagined anything like this period
> of intellectual paralysis. I have been through some kind of
> neurotic experience, curious states… twilight thoughts, veiled
> doubts… The chief patient I am preoccupied with is myself…
> my little hysteria… the analysis is more difficult than any
> other. Something from the deepest depths of my own neurosis
> sets itself against any advance in understanding neuroses…"[79]

According to Freud, hysterical disorders were the result of strong feelings repressed in the subconscious mind, not due to a" strong imagination" or "weak nervous system."

Freud brought the mind back into the body. He thought many essential aspects of our health remain inaccessible to the conscious mind. In his clinical observations, Freud found evidence for the psychological mechanisms of *repression*, a mental device to make the memory of painful or threatening events inaccessible to the conscious mind. He also found evidence for *resistance*, the unconscious mental and emotional defense against awareness of repressed experiences. Through psychotherapy and meditation, we can access some of our unconscious mental processes and release tension from negative emotions.

Freud first used the term "conversion" to refer to the substitution of a somatic (bodily) symptom for a repressed emotion. Thus "conversion disorder" refers to emotional distress or unconscious conflicts which are expressed through physical symptoms—a "mind-body" disorder. Freud (and many others before him) theorized that the disorder may derive from a stressful experience that overwhelmed the patient's psychological and biological coping mechanisms. The emotional conflict was thought to cause the brain to unconsciously disable or impair a bodily function which in turn would prevent the patient from experiencing the stressor again. Conversion disorder can cause a wide-range of motor or sensory deficits, including blindness, seizures or even a temporary form of paralysis.

Freud learned about the bizarre phenomena of hysteria through his mentor, Josef Breuer, who documented hysterical paralysis in his patient, "Anna O." Under hypnosis, "Anna O." began to discuss the circumstances surrounding the onset of her paralysis with Breuer. After several sessions, Breuer discovered that the paralyzed arm was the same arm "Anna O." had used to cradle her dying father and theorized that she was unconsciously halting use of the arm as punishment because she blamed herself for her father's death. She slowly recovered, becoming the "first" successful patient of the "talk cure" or what Freud named "psychoanalysis."

The value of listening to and consoling the patient has been recognized as therapeutic for centuries. Priests, shamans and other "physicians of the soul" promoted healing through emotional catharsis—the ancient Greek ritual of releasing repressed emotions to relieve suffering.[80] The physical brain was so intractable to the late-nineteenth century diagnostics and research modes of investigation that physicians could only theorize about mental functions and behaviors by talking to people. Approaches to the riddles of the human mind were mainly philosophical theories or the creative insights of writers. As a "neuroanatomist," Freud expressed his hope that one day his psychoanalytic theory would be subjected to the scrutiny of science, a hope being realized today through the new science of mind which relies on powerful computers, electron microscopes, imaging technology and experimentation to study the mind. The psychological mechanisms of conversion disorders are still poorly understood today, but like Freud, many physicians believe that the cause is rooted in the subconscious mind.

According to the *Diagnostic and Statistical Manual of Mental Disorders* (DSM), an immediate precipitating source of stress, such as a child's seriousness illness or death, a loss of job or divorce may trigger a *somatoform* illness. The patient may have an unhappy home life or history of sexual or physical abuse. Information from real-time imaging scans, including functional magnetic resonance imaging (fMRI), which measures the brain's use of oxygen during a specific activity; single photon emission computerized tomography (SPECT) and positron emission tomography (PET), which measures the brain's consumption of energy during problem-solving show a dysfunction in the brain's subcortical processes. Brain-scanning also reveals where blood in flowing in tiny groups of neurons and cerebral areas. The healthy brain is able to prevent emotion from interfering with mental functioning through a specific "executive processing" area of the cortex. In conversion disorder, this higher area of reasoning appears inactive on scans, providing a possible clue to the mechanics of the illness. While neurobiological mechanisms may contribute to the condition, brain chemistry doesn't initiate dysfunction—emotions and reason drive neurophysiology that affects bodily sensation and function.

It was also during the late 1800's in which C. G. Jung taught that the psyche was composed of parts, much like the physical body, and Freud made his greatest contribution to science by providing a conceptual framework for the psyche, including the unconscious mind by dividing the mind into *ego, superego* and *id*. According to Freud, the ego or self receives sensory information, processes conscious and unconscious information and interacts with the outside world. The ego also represses instinctual urges from the id, and responds to the pressure of the superego or conscience, the unconscious moral compass of the mind. Freud posited that most mental activity took place below the surface; consciousness was only the "tip of the iceberg." Contemporary neuroscientists now agree: "About 98 percent of what the brain does is outside of conscious awareness," said Michael Gazzaniga.[81]

Physician Walter Cannon first coined the term "fight or flight" to describe physical responses to threats in *Bodily Changes in Pain, Hunger, Fear and Rage: An Account of Recent Researches into the Function of Emotional Excitement* (1915). Cannon revealed the direct relationship between stress and neuroendocrine responses: blood rushes to the skeletal muscles and chemicals flood the nervous system. Cannon believed that brain organized both emotions and bodily arousal. Philosopher and psychologist, William James (1842-1910) thought emotions started in the body and moved up. Experiments performed by neurosurgeon, Wilder Penfield years later showed that both Cannon and James were right: stimulating the limbic region deep in the brain produces simultaneous emotional and physical responses. Communication between the mind and body isn't hierarchical, but simultaneous, rapid and constant. The tight stomach, the tense muscles, the sweaty palms are the emotions, and the emotions are felt throughout the body as sensations.[82] The brain's frontal cortex limits the flow of constant stimuli in order to focus and form our conscious experience. "All our knowledge begins with the senses, proceeds then to the understanding, and ends with reason. There is nothing higher than reason," theorized philosopher Immanuel Kant more than a century before Cannon.

Throughout history, artists, authors, poets and scientists have collaborated to advance both disciplines: Art helps science by providing visual explanations and stimulation of thought; and science helps Art by offering innovative concepts and technological tools that artists can expand into new meanings and insights. Many novelists have captured the fragmented texture of the human mind, including Virginia Woolf, Franz Kafka, Leo Tolstoy, Fyodor Dostoevsky and James Joyce. For example, consider Joyce's third person narration in *The Dead*: "His soul had approached that region where dwell the vast hosts of the dead. He was conscious of, but could not apprehend, their wayward and flickering existence. His own identity was fading out into a grey impalpable world ..."[83] Dostoevsky displayed a nuanced understanding of psychosomatic illness in *Crime and Punishment* (1866). Through the suffering of Raskolnikov, Dostoevsky shows that the body can create real physical symptoms to compensate for deeply repressed emotions such as guilt and fear.

The clinical term "psychosomatic" was coined by pioneering psychiatrist, Helen Flanders Dunbar from the Greek words psyche (mind) and soma (body). In 1935, Dunbar published *Emotions and Bodily Changes: A Survey of Literature on Psychosomatic Interrelationships*, the first modern study on the relationship of emotions to physical disease. Dunbar also established the journal, *Psychosomatic Medicine* and co-founded the American Psychosomatic Society with Franz Alexander in 1942, effectively launching the field. Psychosomatic medicine became popular in the period following World War II when doctors began to see patients with symptoms of post-traumatic stress disorder. Roy R. Grinker's and John P. Spiegel's *Men Under Stress*, an analysis of the psychological stress of warfare and the various therapies used to rehabilitate soldiers, contributed to the popularity of psychosomatic medicine.

Dunbar made the distinction that "psychosomatic" and "imagined" were not synonymous. The symptoms experienced from psychosomatic illness are as real as the symptoms experienced from an organic illness but the mechanisms beneath the illnesses are different.

Psychosomatic disorders are defined as any physical disorders induced or modified by the brain for psychological reasons. Powerful unconscious emotions are responsible for psychosomatic disorders. Psychosomatic medicine was in its heyday when psychoanalyst Alexander published *Psychosomatic Medicine* in 1950.

The emotion underlying most psychosomatic illnesses is *stress*—a factor all too prevalent during the first half of the twentieth century, during the Cold War and post-9/11. One of the most comprehensive definitions of "stress" can be found in Brian Seaward's *Essentials of Managing Stress*:

> Stress is the inability to cope with a *perceived* (real or imagined) threat to one's mental, physical, emotional, and spiritual well-being, which results in a series of physiological responses and adaptations.[84]

Stress is an interaction between a person and the environment. It's not just a function of what's out there—it's a function of how the person is dealing with what's out there.

Psychologist Franz Alexander believed that chronic stress led to tissue changes in various organs, eventually causing disease, and drew connections between specific personality types and diseases like asthma and hypertension, a theory that contemporary research supports. Researchers have correlated activity in the emotion-processing centers of the brain to inflammatory mechanisms known to influence asthma and a spectrum of conditions associated with aging, including cardiovascular disease, osteoporosis, arthritis, type-2 diabetes mellitus, and certain cancers.[85] According to Esther Sternberg, M.D., a NIH senior scientist, "It is ironic that research into infectious and inflammatory disease first led twentieth century medicine to reject the idea that the mind influences physical illness, and now research in the same field … is proving contrary."[86]

The American faith in the power of the individual to reinvent him or herself was a popular movement in the late nineteenth century and into the 1960's and even somewhat today. According to medical historian, Anne Harrington:

> William James took an active and supportive interest in what he called "The Religion of Healthy-Mindedness" which, he

reported in 1902, 'has recently poured over America and seems to be gathering force every day.' James claimed that 'mind-cure gives to some of us serenity, moral poise, and happiness, and prevents certain forms of disease as well as science does, or even better in a certain class of persons.[87]

From Ralph Waldo Emerson's "Self-Reliance," Dale Carnegie's *How to Win Friends and Influence People* to today's spiritually-based liberalism of U2's Bono and more conservative Christians who are aspiring to be born again—that faith in the power of the individual to transform continues to be present in our culture and nation. "I celebrate myself," Walt Whitman sang in his "Song of Myself." As Willy Loman, perhaps the archetype of American self-reinvention puts it in Arthur Miller's *Death of a Salesman*, "A man can't go out the way he came in, Ben, he has got to add up to something." Being proactive about your health is big business. Consider the international popularity of Lance Armstrong after defeating brain cancer and winning the Tour de France. Or take a look at the stacks of self-help books in your local library or bookstore with titles such as Norman Cousin's *The Anatomy of an Illness* and Wayne Sotile's Thriving with *Heart Disease*.

Positive emotions can help keep a person's chemical and neural responses in balance, and help people handle stress better, but it would be a great disservice to my patients, doctors and the public if this book were misconstrued to imply that "self-help" tactics such as putting on a happy face or seeking an emotional catharsis will keep brain or breast cancer at bay. Does chronic stress contribute to acute or chronic infection? For decades doctors believed that stress caused ulcers and were slow to prescribe antibiotics for them until 1984, when two Australians, Dr. Barry J. Marshall and Dr. J. Robin Warren, identified H. pylori among ulcer patients. Researchers only recently discovered that millions of women (and fewer men) have a form of heart disease that may not be detected with standard diagnostics—tiny blocked arterioles in the heart. For years women with chest pain and normal coronary arteries were told that their symptoms were related to anxiety.

Disease typically but not always has recognizable signs and a known cause, such as a necrotizing tumor within the breast. Hidden neurological lesions are rare, perhaps only one out of every five-hundred cases, but I can think of one case I've seen in the last five years: Angie, a recently married, 23 year old redhead with sensitive tailbone pain and no previous injury. She had seen several specialists, including a neurologist, orthopedist and psychiatrist. The only test not done was a CT scan of the sacrum, a triangular bone at the base of the spine that joins to the hip bone on either side of the pelvis. The scan revealed that she had a benign neurofibroma (tumor) of the sacrum and surgery cured her. A misdiagnosis, failed surgery or a dismissive doctor can be profoundly disillusioning to the patient, or worse. Doctors are hard-wired to make sense of the world, and that includes both rational and irrational assumptions influenced by the culture of a given time period. Human reasoning is plagued by problems that include personal prejudices, overdependence on authority, overemphasis on coincidence, distortion of the evidence and circular reasoning. "Man thinks, God laughs," (a Yiddish aphorism).

In my experience, the true cause of pain and illness are often unknown, and sometimes relate to the more subjective aspects of human beings. Psychosomatic medicine, specifically the Freudian-based theories related to the unconscious, provide a conceptual framework that can help doctors and patients understand that psychology, not physiology is often the root of many chronic illnesses such as back pain. Our immune system can be activated or inhibited by emotional states and our attitudes and beliefs about what is occurring to us. To the extent that perceived stress contributes to disease or illness, the self-initiated solution is more subtle and arduous, and partly has to do with cultivating emotional intelligence, or what Daniel Goleman defines as, "self-awareness, seeing the links between thoughts, feelings and reactions; knowing if thoughts or feelings are ruling a decision; seeing the consequence of alternative choices; and applying these insights to choices."[88] Part genetic predisposition, part life experience, and part old-fashioned common sense and hard work, emotional intelligence emerges in varying degrees from person to person.

Having emotional intelligence means coping with stress without losing control or turning to food, alcohol or drug abuse. It also means recognizing the intuitive power of emotions, what Aristotle viewed as a source of wisdom and perception during times of adversity. A primary method for gaining emotional intelligence is to do what Norman Vincent Peale recommended to Americans decades ago: practice emptying the mind. Researchers say the biological effects of meditation—the production of antibodies against illness and the general sense of well-being—last up to four months after the end of meditation training.[89] Recognize that unconscious and conscious emotions, thoughts and beliefs can affect reality. Contemporary physician John Sarno has had tremendous success in relieving chronic back pain by treating what he believes is the psychological and emotional basis to the illness. To heal means "to make whole." In my experience, treating the chemistry of many chronic disorders doesn't cure them. The best medical therapy combines conventional medicine with self-initiated activities that exercise the body; practice good nutrition; and cultivate psychological insights, such as meditation (even golf can be a form of meditation), psychoanalysis or reading.

Researchers at Johns Hopkins reported that cancer patients who showed a "fighting spirit," tended to live longer than did those who were passive and "good." Scientists began to follow a group of 36 women who had been diagnosed as having advanced breast cancer. After seven years, 24 of the 36 women had died. The only psychological factor that mattered for survival within seven years seemed to be a sense of joy with life. The primary factor that predicted survival was already well established in oncology: the length of time the patients remained disease-free after first being treated, and before having a relapse. But the second-strongest factor was having a high score on "joy" on a standard paper-and-pencil test measuring mood. Test evidence of joy was statistically more significant as a predictor of survival than was the number of sites of metastases once the cancer spread. That a joyous state of mind should be so powerful a predictor of survival was completely unexpected.

Perhaps the most important contribution of Freud, Alexander and Dunbar was the recognition that pain and illness could be psychogenic— physical symptoms could originate in the subconscious mind. Today host of functional, non-organic disorders have replaced the hysteria, neurasthenia and psychosomatic diagnoses of the past: post-traumatic stress disorder (PTSD), tension myositis (TMS), fibromyalgia, chronic fatigue syndrome (CFS), panic attacks, inappropriate sinus tachycardia (IST), irritable bowel syndrome (IBS,) vasovagal or neurocardiogenic syncope, and postural orthostatic tachycardia syndrome (POTS). Many questions about functional disorders remain unanswered, but research has begun to suggest how chronic emotional stress may alter the function of normal sensory, pain and motor circuits in the brain, immune, endocrine and nervous systems.

Integrative health physicians, including Andrew Weil often attribute panic attacks, inappropriate sinus tachycardia (IST) and neurocardiogenic syncope to a poorly understood autonomic nervous system (ANS) imbalance related to the body's "fight or flight" response. The ANS controls the body's unconscious stress response—blood pressure, heart rate, digestion, and breathing patterns. Exercise, yoga, tai-chi, massage therapy, and stretching therapy can counter ANS disorders by balancing the biological affects of chronic stress. When stress persists for a long time, and the body is chronically overactive, immune resistance fails and the body moves to the exhaustion stage. In this stage, the body is vulnerable to disease and even death.

Dunbar hoped that psychosomatic medicine would integrate the treatment of spiritual, emotional and physical suffering into a single framework versus symptom-centered treatments.[90] Such treatments refer to medical care that focuses on immediate results without regard for the root cause. Dunbar emphasized treating the patient as a complete individual, following the Hippocratic tenet that: "It is more important to know what sort of person has a disease than to know what sort of disease a person has." Somewhere along the long line of medicine's successive evolution, doctors lost sight of the whole patient, and focus instead on fighting the agent of disease and illness—the bacterial microbe, fungus or toxin. As Susan Sontag notes in *Illness as Metaphor*, disease is now seen as an invasion of alien organisms, to which the body responds by its own military operations, such as the mobilizing of immunological "defenses," and medicine is "aggressive," as in the language of most chemotherapies. [91]

In my line of specialty medicine, there is a tendency to see pain and illness in purely mechanical terms. Medical diagnosis must involve taking the time to get to know the patient, especially in the clinical setting of surgery where lives are potentially at stake. The clinical objectivity that enters into medical decision-making must be combined with knowledge of the psyche, Hippocratic ethics, and holistic values to have the greatest impact on healing and recovery. "Where love of mankind is, there is also love of the Art," said Hippocrates in his *Precepts*.

PART II

The Fundamental Unity
of Mind and Body

CHAPTER 4

The Bridge between Mind and Body

A sad soul can kill you quicker than a germ.

–John Steinbeck

After the invention of the hypodermic needle in the mid-nineteenth century, morphine replaced the use of raw opium for medical purposes and became the standard intravenous painkiller. Scientists and doctors didn't know how morphine worked, but they theorized people had to produce something in the body that could "receive" the drug's molecules in order to produce its pharmacological effects.

No one had ever found such an internal "receptor" until Candace Pert, Ph.D. discovered the opiate receptor in 1972. Pert and her team at the NIH used an innovative photographic technique called "autoradiography" that uses radioactive materials and high power microscopy to detect and map the microscopic pathways of cells and molecules in the brain. Use of this technique unveiled a chemical brain: cell receptors could be seen as sparkling grains in an area of stained brain tissue. Her ground-breaking discovery revealed how powerful pain-relieving drugs like morphine and heroin affect the brain, and introduced an important new method for studying the molecular biochemistry of the mind.

The first molecular revolution in science took place in 1953 when James Watson and Francis Crick proposed the double helix model for DNA, opening the door to the individual properties of living matter, cells. The discovery of the opiate receptor and opioids sparked a second molecular revolution, reviving neuroscience. Academic labs, pharmaceutical-company research departments, and scientific institutes around the world began to quantify the biochemistry that influences the mind. By the end of the twentieth century, scientists had mapped the human body's extraordinary system of receptors, tiny sensing devices that initiate the action of biochemicals in the brain and body.

"On a cellular level," explains neuroscientist Dr. Pert, "receptors are our eyes, ears and nose waiting to pick up signals." Receptors are molecules, the smallest possible piece of a substance. Receptor molecules respond to energy and chemical cues by vibrating. They "wiggle, shimmy, and even hum" as they bend and change from one shape to another under the microscope. Every living human cell is studded with hundreds of thousands of receptors. "Think of them as lily pads floating on the surface of a pond."[92] A brain cell may have millions of receptors on its surface.

Receptors cluster in the membrane of cells "dancing and vibrating" until the right chemical keys swim up and mount them by fitting into their keyholes—a process known as *binding* (or sex on a molecular level). Receptors bind with specific types of molecules called "ligands" (binding agents) through a vibratory force that produces a reverberating pitch like a tuning fork. After binding with a ligand, the receptor releases information deep inside the cell where the "message" changes the state of the cell dramatically. A cascade of biochemical events follows. These minute physiological changes influence the mood, behavior, movement and immunity of living organisms. Our emotional states result from turning certain molecular activity on while turning others off. For example, fear in response to danger activates the sympathetic nervous system and depresses the gastrointestinal tract and sexual organs.

Discovering the opiate receptor led to a race to find the substance in the brain that binds with it, a scientific competition that culminated with the discovery of endogenous opioids—the body's own natural morphine or "endorphins." Psychoactive drugs such as morphine work because they mimic natural endorphins. They bind to the same receptors but can have more extreme effects on mood, blood pressure and breathing. In response to long-term use of morphine, the brain creates "pseudo" receptors for endorphins. Abstaining from morphine allows the brain to gradually replace bogus receptors with functioning ones.

Receptors for endorphins can be found all over the body—in organs, tissues, blood and bones. Endorphins help regulate such vital functions as hunger, thirst, mood, immune response, cardiac and vascular function and other involuntary or subconscious physiological processes. A concentration of opiate receptors exists in the respiratory center, serving as a kind of metronome regulating breathing according to the body's requirements. The digestive system inhibits intestinal movements through opioids. Even the heart has opiate receptors for signals the brain sends to the heart. (The heart actually sends more signals to the brain than the brain sends to the heart).

Human Cell with Ligand-Receptor Interactions

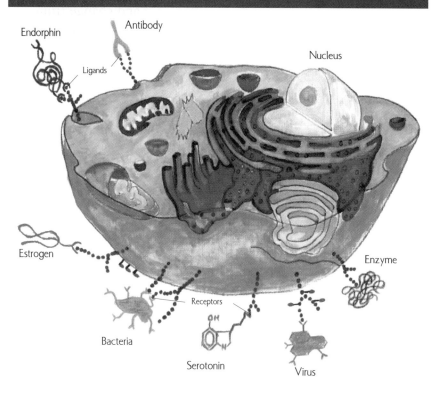

FIGURE 2: The body contains an extraordinary system of receptors, tiny sensing devices that initiate a chain reaction of biochemicals. On a cellular level, receptors are our eyes, ears and nose waiting to pick up signals. Every living human cell is studded with hundreds of thousands of receptors. Receptors bind with specific types of molecules called ligands through a vibratory force. After binding with a ligand, the receptor releases information deep inside the cell where the "message" changes the state of the cell.

When scientists discovered endorphins in the immune system, they had to repeat their experiments several times before anyone would believe them. Endorphins help reduce pain during infection, inflammation and swelling. They also eliminate pain during shock, the intense physiological state of collapse related to sudden physical or emotional trauma such as an automobile accident. The rush of endorphins during a stressful event creates nausea. Finding receptors for endorphins on white blood cells provided biological evidence that confirms the conventional wisdom: sickness influences emotions.

After the discovery of endorphins, researchers began to map the anatomical architecture of emotional expression in specific structures of the brain, and discovered a dense distribution of opiate receptors in the brain's limbic system, a group of brain structures that play a role in emotion. Endorphins are peptides, a class of informational substances called "ligands" that act as messengers between cells in the brain and throughout the body.

The "Second Nervous System"

The ligand-receptor system functions as a "second nervous system" that communicates across great lengths of the body through nerve pathways or the bloodstream, and like the central nervous system has a fundamental role in the control of behavior. Ligands are any natural or manmade substance that binds selectively to a specific receptor on the surface of a cell. They vary in size and critical function and have a powerful influence on states of mind. The three basic types of ligands and some of their better-known sub-types include:
- Neurotransmitters (acetylcholine, norepinephrine, dopamine, serotonin)
- Hormones (estrogen, testosterone, progesterone, cortisol)
- Peptides (oxytocin, ACTH, CRH, vasopressin, opioids)

Neurotransmitters are small molecules that carry information across the synaptic bridge between one neuron and the next. Activation of the neurotransmitter acetylcholine increases your concentration, focus and memory but in large concentrations can cause agitation. Nicotine binds to the receptor for acetylcholine. Pleasurable actions such as eating, drinking or sex can increase levels of the neurotransmitter, dopamine. People experiencing depression or anxiety may have a dopamine deficiency. Many drugs of abuse that give people pleasurable or calming highs, such as cocaine, appear to work by mimicking dopamine. Serotonin has various functions in the human body including the control of appetite, sleep, memory and learning, temperature regulation, mood, behavior, cardiovascular function, muscle contraction, endocrine regulation and depression. The action of neurotransmitters can be overdone or shut down by the ingestion of drugs, poor nutrition, viruses or bacteria, aging and stress.

Hormones are produced in nearly every organ system and tissue in the body. The best-known hormones are testosterone and estrogen. Hormones guide sexual, reproductive, nurturing and aggressive behaviors in men and women. In *The Female Brain*, neuroscientist

Louann Brizendine writes that hormones have massive neurological effects on men and women at different stages of life, shaping desires, values and the way we perceives reality. Peptides are the largest category of ligands, and perhaps make-up most of the conversation between brain and body.

Your body has more than an estimated 100 peptides aiding in digestion, breathing and many other functions—they can affect gene expression, the formation of new connections between brain cells, and other vital cellular changes. Peptides play a huge role in regulating all life processes. "If the cell is the engine that drives all life, then the receptors are the buttons on the control panel of that engine, and a specific ligand (a peptide 95 percent of the time) is the finger that pushes that button and gets things started."[93] Peptides are produced inside our cells and released into the surrounding fluids, then recycled back into the building blocks of amino acids. Enzymes on the surface of every single cell will destroy peptides quickly after their release. In contrast, the liver metabolizes and excretes exogenous (artificial) drugs like morphine over a period of many hours.

The nervous, endocrine, cardiovascular, digestive and immune systems are interlocked in a body-wide system where each part can communicate with every other part through signaling molecules. Many different kinds of brain messengers exist in the brain and throughout the body. Individual amino acids such as GABA transmit many messages to the brain. Neuropeptides are heavier molecules and slower-acting than neurotransmitters. Neuropeptides can act in concert with a neurotransmitter, but their signals play a different role. They tend to have more prolonged influences and striking effects on mood, personality and human behavior by affecting gene expression. For example, dense amounts of mu-opioid receptors are found in the frontal cortex, the brain structure unique to humans in the animal kingdom. The stimulation of mu-opioids in the brain creates a powerful sense of bliss, serenity and analgesia. This was the first clue to the emotional aspect of receptor physiology. Second messengers associated with the receptors are primed to learn and reward certain behaviors such as feeding.

The new view of the chemical mind began to turn science upside down during the latter half of the twentieth century, increasing the role and promise of the pharmaceutical industry as scientists began uncovering the chemical processes that trigger our immunology, moods, behaviors and beliefs. Today psychology is no longer considered the only gateway to the mind; a multidisciplinary research approach exists between biochemistry, molecular biophysics, genetics, neurology and psychology.

The discovery of a dense amount of neuropeptides in the emotional part of the brain led scientists to theorize that neuropeptides form the biochemical basis of emotion. Scientists can't look at a particular neuropeptide under the microscope, so to speak, and name the emotion. "Look, here's sadness. Or that's anger." According to this view, emotions are the nexus or communication vehicle between mind and body, going back and forth between the two and influencing both.

Charles Darwin speculated that emotions must be the key to survival of the fittest. His book, *Expressions of Emotions in Man and Animals*, explains how people everywhere have common emotional expressions, some shared by animals. One of Darwin's hypotheses was that opiate receptors are found throughout evolution from a single cell. Experiments have proven just that—opiate receptors exist throughout the vertebral brains of living creatures, from snails and jellyfish to gorillas and giraffes. Even insects have opiate receptors, although the thought of a fly with feelings disturbs me. Eric Kandel in his book, *In Search of Memory* cites the biological retention of information molecules as a key principle in the new science of mind.

How Emotions Influence Immunity

Ancient Greek physicians held that whatever happens in the mind influences the body, and vice versa. But the wisdom of the ages lacked the tools to prove the biochemistry between mind, body and health. Today scientists know that several different neural and chemical pathways link the brain and immune system, the body's loosely organized defense system that responds automatically to any foreign invader. A central discovery was that monocytes manufacture neuropeptides, proving a two-way communication system between the brain and the immune system.

The central nervous and immune systems are similar in their modes of receiving, recognizing, and interpreting stimuli from the environment but the immune system operates as a decentralized network. Your immune system can trigger emotions that motivate behavior. A key property of immune cells is that they move. Peptides can control the routing and secretion of monocytes and communicate with other lymphocytes—B and T cells—by interacting through cytokines, lymphokines and interleukins to launch a well-coordinated attack anywhere in the body.

Discoveries within the past few decades suggest many specific interactions of a similar kind between the brain and immune defenses. Hormones and molecules released by the nervous system can affect the immune system and vice versa. That is, the brain's messages to hormone-producing glands and the circulatory system affect the immune system; in turn, activity of the immune defenses, directly or indirectly, influences the brain. Every neuropeptide known to exist in the brain and spinal cord also exist on the surface of the immune system's monocytes. Monocytes, cells in the immune system that act to heal wounds, repair tissue and ingest bacteria and other foreign bodies, also manufacture neuropeptides that communicate with the body and the brain, influencing emotions and immunity. A very high concentration of receptors for neuropeptides exists in the brainstem, the part of the brain that regulates the autonomic nervous system (ANS) associated with involuntary bodily functions.

The science that links stress, the immune system and disease has more questions than answers, but concrete evidence proves biochemical links between hormones in the body and cells in the immune system and brain. Psychological experiences, such as stress and anxiety, can influence immune function, which in turn may have an effect on the course of disease and illness. The immune system, research suggests, is one source of the chemicals that, in the brain, control mood to marshal energy elsewhere.

While studying taste aversion in mice at Indiana University in 1981, neuroanatomist Robert Ader and his team discovered that the immune system can be conditioned in the same way Pavlov's dogs learned to salivate in response to a bell. In their study, mice prone to Lupus were offered a saccharin-flavored drink at the same time they were injected with a potent immunosuppressive drug to treat their inflammatory disease. Once the association was learned, the taste alone (with no injection at all) reduced inflammation and symptoms of Lupus almost as much as the drug alone. The experiment proved that the immune system can be conditioned just like the mind: the immune system can learn. Ader and his team also found nerves in the thymus and spleen terminating near clusters of lymphocytes, macrophages, and mast cells, all of which help control immune function. If nerves from the spleen or lymph nodes were removed, the immune responses didn't function.[94] The discovery demonstrated that the brain is capable of exerting regulation over the immune system and visa versa.

More recent studies show that the activity of certain immune defense cells called "natural killer cells" can be greatly enhanced by the brain's trained response to a totally extraneous stimulus from the outside world—a strong odor. The killer cells are part of the body's surveillance system that protects against invasion and possibly against cancer.[95] Study of the links between the mind, brain and immune system is called psychoneuroimmunology.

Full Circle

Until Candace Pert discovered the opiate receptor laying the groundwork for a new method of studying molecular biology, a brain-centered view of emotions was the prevailing wisdom of Western science. Neuropharmacology focused on neurotransmitters released from nerve endings, traveling across synapses and passing information along that effects mental activity and behavior. The process involves billions of synaptic connections between billions of neurons. The electrical and chemical brain seemed to merge at the synapse. Renowned NIH neuroscientist Miles Herkenham estimated that, counter to the collective wisdom of neuropharmacologists and neuroscientists, *less than 20 percent* of neuronal communication actually occurs at the synapse. The possible lines of communication between the brain and body are numerous.

Scientists in the latter half of the twentieth century presented new theories of information outside the bounds of the nervous system, focusing on purely chemical, non-synaptic communication between cells. For example, Pert and her research team systemically analyzed brain distribution patterns of thirty-three different neuropeptide receptors and compared them to the classical brain location of the limbic system. They found that core limbic brain structures contained a whopping *85-95 percent* of the neuropeptide receptors. The implications were that emotions are primarily chemical. A new way of thinking about the brain emerged: researchers determined that the brain is kept in order not only by synaptic connections of brain cells,

Neuron Communication

MACRO VIEW

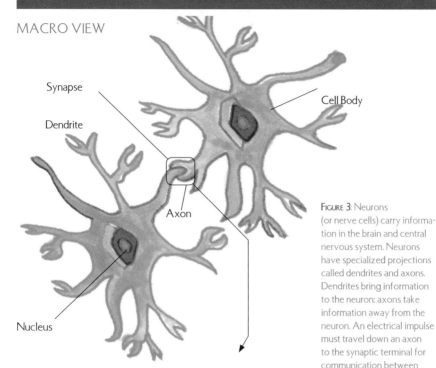

Synapse

Dendrite

Cell Body

Axon

Nucleus

FIGURE 3: Neurons (or nerve cells) carry information in the brain and central nervous system. Neurons have specialized projections called dendrites and axons. Dendrites bring information to the neuron; axons take information away from the neuron. An electrical impulse must travel down an axon to the synaptic terminal for communication between neurons to occur.

MICRO VIEW

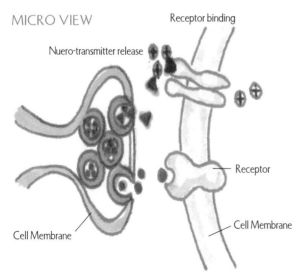

Receptor binding

Nuero-transmitter release

Receptor

Cell Membrane

Cell Membrane

SIGNAL-EMITTING NEURON

SIGNAL-RECEIVING NEURON

Information from one neuron flows to another neuron across a small gap called a synapse. All messages are passed between connected neurons in the form of tiny molecules called neurotransmitters. They flow from a signal-emitting neuron across the synapse and bind with receptors on the surface of the signal-receiving neuron. The binding action triggers a chain of chemical reactions within the cell's nucleus that can alter states of mind. The brain keeps tight control of this message delivery system; disruption leads to susceptibility to disease and illness.

but by the specificity of the receptors, or in other words, the ability of the receptors to bind only with one kind of ligand.

Studies soon demonstrated that the autonomic nervous system contained almost every neuropeptide. New peptide-containing groups of cells called "nuclei," the source of brain-body and body-brain hook-ups, were also discovered. At this juncture in science, Freud would announce (if he were alive): "The body is the subconscious mind."[96]

Biochemical changes wrought on the receptor level is the molecular basis of memory. The fact that memory is encoded or stored at the receptor level means that memory processes are emotion-driven and unconscious. Repressed emotions are stored in the body—your subconscious mind—via the release of neuropeptic ligands. The memories are in the receptors. According to one theory on illness, when the subconscious mind tries to relieve itself of this increasing subconscious turmoil, there is a limit and severe mind-body illnesses develop. Type II Diabetes, for example, seems to be associated with defective receptors, allowing glucose to build up in the blood by blocking the path of insulin, the type of ligand called a peptide that binds with receptors on muscle and fat cells.[97]

Modern scientists have begun to prove the chemistry and anatomy behind the mind-body, body-mind network. Research on neuropeptides demonstrated that the brain is not just an electrical organ, but a neuropeptide network with a two-way system of communication with the body. Neuropeptides perform about 90 percent of the work of peptides, forming a vast long-distance communication system between the mind and body, body and mind.

Cells in the immune system that act to heal wounds, repair tissue and ingest bacteria and other foreign invaders are shaped in such a way that they invite chemical interaction with neuropeptides. If you recall, neuropeptides serve as chemical messengers between brain cells, and also regulate organs. A particularly strong concentration of immune cells interacts with neuropeptides in the limbic system, the network of brain structures that controls emotion. Moreover, the immune system itself, research suggests, is one source of the chemicals that, in the brain, control mood.

A blood-brain barrier forms between cerebral blood vessels and brain tissue to keep out foreign invaders such as bacteria. For years, scientists thought the immune system could not communicate with the brain due to the tight security system. Today we know that immune cytokines, such as IL-1 receptors, can bind on cells lining cerebral blood vessels to trigger prostaglandin-producing enzymes and cause fever. The binding also triggers other enzymes that produce gases such as nitric oxide. These molecules are small enough to penetrate the blood-brain barrier and signal brain cells to produce hormones that cause sickness behaviors.

A key property of the immune system is that it moves throughout the body. The emotion-generating peptides control the routing and secretion of monocytes and communicate with other immune cells called lymphocytes—B and T cells—by interacting through peptides called cytokines, lymphokines and interleukins. Thus the immune system can launch a well-coordinated attack against disease.

The practical implication is that the many stresses in life impact the immune system. The final cure for cancer will probably be increasing your immunity. Until recently, many scientists and physicians were skeptical that the brain-immune communication was real and questioned whether it had any relevance to human disease. A 1987 article in *The New England Journal of Medicine* even called it "folklore." In response to this, one of the field's key researchers, Esther Sternberg, set out to convince academics that there was substantial research proving that the brain and immune systems do communicate and that this communication plays a very important part in health and disease.

Sternberg's book *The Balance Within: The Science Connecting Health and Emotions* explores the science of the mind-body connection, the reasons this field was at first rejected by the academic scientific community and how it has come *full circle* to acceptance. Many medical textbooks now feature chapters on the brain-immune connection in health and disease. This work does not address psychological conditions or stress, but shows that an impaired hormonal stress response is associated with inflammatory disease. Your brain plays an important role in translating thoughts, attitude and emotions into nerve energy and biochemistry—but peptides play an even larger role. The thoughts and emotions that seem to color our reality are the result of complex electrochemical interactions within and between nerve cells.

Research into stem cells generated in bone marrow has revealed their remarkable ability to become different types of cells, including immune cells. In 2000, researchers studying brain tissue from patients

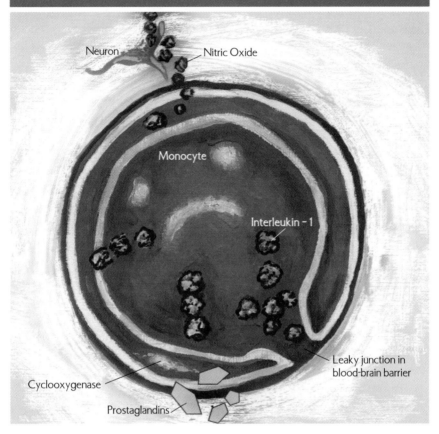

Cerebral Blood Vessel and Immune System Interactions

Neuron

Nitric Oxide

Monocyte

Interleukin – 1

Leaky junction in
blood-brain barrier

Cyclooxygenase

Prostaglandins

FIGURE 4: Endothelial cells lining cerebral blood vessels form a tight "blood-brain barrier" to protect the brain from bacteria and other pathogens. During the immune system's response to infection or irritation, cytokines, small proteins secreted by the lymph system, such as Interleukin-1 bind with receptors on the endothelial cells to trigger a series of molecular reactions. Enzymes, including cyclooxygenase produce molecules of prostaglandins that signal neurons to cause fever. Other enzymes synthesize nitric oxide to signal neurons to produce hormones that cause lethargy, malaise and loss of appetite. Cytokines can escape through leaky junctions in the blood-brain barrier near the hypothalamus and bind with neurons to activate the brain's stress center.

who died after bone marrow transplants provided evidence that stem cells can migrate to the brain and blossom into clumps of active gray and white matter. According to Eva Mezey, M.D. from the National Institute of Neurological Disorders and Stroke (NINDS), "Adult stem cells could some day be used to replace neural elements lost to neurodegenerative diseases, stroke, or trauma." A new protocol replaces dying brain cells in Parkinson disease with stem cells, easing symptoms in a rat model of the disease, but also raises the concern that poorly differentiated cells have the potential to become cancerous. "We need to determine how cells in the blood enter the brain, how to induce them to enter the brain in larger numbers, how to promote their differentiation into neurons and how to target them to areas of need."[98] Mezey's discovery more deeply connects the brain to the body, proving once again, all is one.

Brain and Immune System Communication

Figure 5

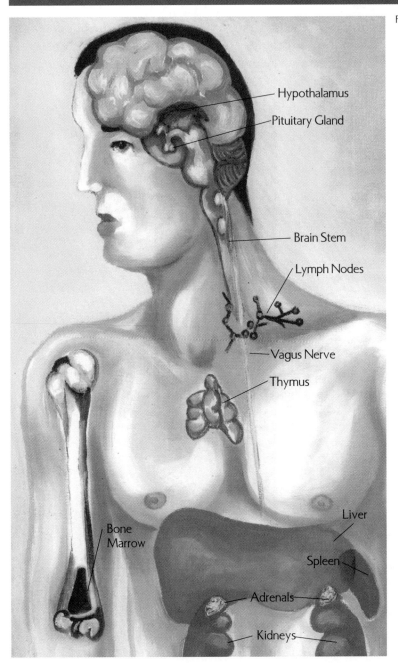

Hypothalamus

Pituitary Gland

Brain Stem

Lymph Nodes

Vagus Nerve

Thymus

Liver

Bone Marrow

Spleen

Adrenals

Kidneys

Brain and Immune System Communication Cont.

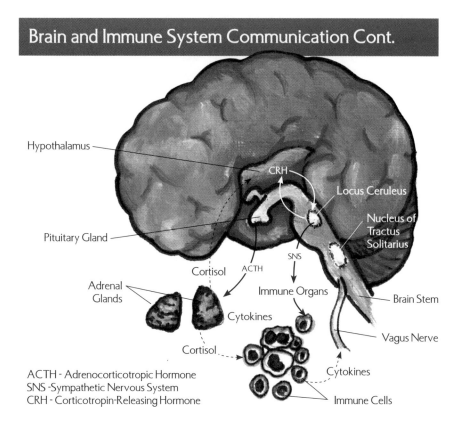

Figure 6: The immune system has a diffuse and dynamic defense network involving the spleen, thymus, lymph nodes, and bone marrow. A threatening situation triggers the brain's hypothalamus to secrete corticotrophin-releasing hormone (CRH) which in turn stimulates the pituitary gland to secrete adrenocorticotropin hormone (ACTH). ACTH signals the adrenal glands (located above each kidney) to release cortisol, the hormone that modulates the body's "fight or flight" response. Cortisol also balances the stress response by acting on the hypothalamus to inhibit the continued release of CRH.

The immune system can signal the brain through tiny proteins called cytokines that activate the vagus nerve or travel through the bloodstream. In turn, the brain can regulate the immune system through neurotransmitters and hormones such as cortisol.

Perpetual activation of the stress response can damage healthy cells and weaken the immune system. IgA (immunoglobulin A) is an immune system antibody and one of the body's first lines of defense against colds, flu and infections of the respiratory and urinary tracts. IgA is found in our saliva, lungs, digestive and urinary systems. A single episode of stress, anger or frustration can depress the level of IgA in your immune system for almost an entire day.

CHAPTER 5

Brain Fallacies

Death may be aging, but he still has clout.

–Harold Pinter

One early April evening while on trauma duty, I received a call that a seventeen-year-old boy had arrived in the Emergency Room due to a motorcycle accident. I was watching the evening news with my family. The Chernobyl reactor was open to the sky and burning, sending a plume of radioactive smoke into the atmosphere. After talking on the phone with the attending physician for several minutes, I asked my daughter and the co-author of this book, Kim, to join me on my trip to the hospital.

The spring air was cold. When we arrived at Parkview Memorial Hospital, I exchanged my suit jacket for a white coat and escorted Kim down the dim-lit hallway of the Intensive Care Unit. Lights and sounds are kept low in the ICU bay to promote sedation. I opened a sliding glass door into a sanitized room where green and orange monitor lights were flashing. David, a seventeen-year-old with a bandaged forehead, was intubated, ventilated and restrained to the side-rails of the hospital bed. The restraints were necessary to prevent injuries from seizures due to brain swelling. An IV line was running into his arm.

Standing at David's bedside, I bent over and lifted his eyelids with my thumb. Wide black pupils stared back, fixed and dilated as the attending physician had noted. I felt my stomach drop. Despite advanced operative techniques and technology, I knew I couldn't save him. David was past the point of surgery. I turned to my teenage daughter to see her reaction. She understood. Until now, I felt like I was doing the right thing by asking her to come. But now I wasn't so sure. Her blue eyes were sullen. Disassociation and denial, the ability to squash your own emotions and compartmentalize was my job requirement, not hers. I walked over to where Kim was standing and put my arm around her.

David's impending death sent ripples through the ICU. Nurses, orderlies and physicians came and went from the room. His boyish face was ashen and sweaty. There was no obvious bruising or Battle's sign yet, a bruise found below the ear suggesting fracture of the base of the skull. At first glance, the head bandage was ennobling, a perverted crown on his youth, cut off like a flower. I put on a sterile latex glove and carefully lifted the gauze. The accident had fractured his skull and scalped the crown of his forehead. Skin flapped open. Blood ran down his face. I covered him back up.

David was a powerfully built teenager with a broad chest and muscular arms and legs. The length of his body filled the bed. He was a junior in high school and rugby player who I recognized from the "Sports" section of the *Fort Wayne Journal Gazette*. Riding his motorcycle without a helmet down Interstate 69, David hit a slick spot and skid head-first into a car. He arrived in the ER at about 7:00 pm with an open head injury and severe traumatic brain injury. As I listened to his accelerated heart rate with my stethoscope, the door slid open again and my nurse, Diana, told me that the boy's parents were on the way. With one glance she took in the scene. The dying brain has distinct external signs. Enzymes break-down tissue causing cellular death and making the brain soft and malleable, which means it can shift into intracranial spaces and force cerebrospinal fluid where it does *not* belong, like the ear canals. Diana began to prepare David for his family. She wiped his bloody face and liquid draining from his ears. My daughter turned and stared out the window.

Earlier that year, Kim bought a Yamaha DT 250 at college and rode the 180 miles of interstate and highways between Bloomington and Fort Wayne, Indiana without a helmet. When she arrived at our house, she hid the motorcycle in the alleyway behind our garage. From the perspective of a parent, her behavior was enraging. Today I understand how my daughter could make such decisions. Neuroscience now knows that the frontal cortex, the region in the brain critical to good decision-making, develops late in adolescence. This is why parents need to help adolescents make decisions and change behavior that threatens their lives, health or safety.

After Diana left and we were alone again with David, I turned to Kim and said, "Severe trauma to the brain causes irreversible liquid necrosis. The brain literally turns to mush." She looked away. "You see? *Do you see*, Kim? This seventeen-year-old boy will not walk out of here. It's a fallacy of your age to think you're invincible." Clinical practice has toughened my heart but hasn't closed my mind to novel ways of creating lasting impressions.

I resumed my neurological exam and pressed the red call button to ask Diana to repack his head wound, increase the rate of the ventilator, and administer the drug mannitol to reduce intracranial pressure. I wanted to buy some time. David's parents arrived within minutes. I went out to the lobby to meet them, leaving my daughter behind at the busy nurse's station.

Diana pointed to a couple standing in the crowded hallway, indicating to me that they were David's parents. A circle of hospital staff surrounded them. I approached slowly yet purposely and said, "Hello, I'm Dr. Rudy Kachmann."

David's mother let go of her husband's arm to shake my hand. She was tall and athletic looking, her eyes were wide and alert, scanning my face.

I turned to the father and extended my hand to him.

"How does it look, doctor?" There was more fear than despair in his question. The father asked, shaking my hand. His thick eyebrows weighed heavily over his eyes. His gold-rimmed glasses were smudged.

I took them into a private room with a lamp, comfortable chairs and carpeting. A Bible sat on the table. And then I sat down, leaned forward and said what I've had to say more than once, but never when it had such personal relevance. "This is a terrible, *terrible* situation …" my voice broke. I couldn't look another parent in the eye and say what I fear most without feeling it in my heart. I told them that David was brain-dead. The chance that an unresponsive, severely brain-damaged patient would recover depends on the type of injury suffered and on the length of time he or she has been unresponsive. I explained why in David's case, our neurosurgical options were null, and recommended to withdraw life-support when they were ready to do so. They were overcome, crying and struggling to ask questions. I offered to meet with them the next morning and afternoon, and any day, any time after that. I also told them about my daughter's own motorcycle. The mother nodded. I could see the pulse in her neck throbbing beneath the skin. I took her hand in mine and held it for long seconds as she began to shake and sob.

Deeper Than the Knife

Every patient, every *person* can learn new ways to cope with the common maladies of our human condition: vague terrorist warnings, vehicular traffic and road rage, unstable jobs and marriages, parental anxiety, depression, isolation and loneliness. That is, everyone needs emotional care, some more than others at different times in their lives. I've found that people are often better equipped to overcome illness or surgery when their needs are met by a caring, empathetic listener, such as a physician, friend, counselor or spiritual advisor. Emotional intuition is a blind spot for many doctors. Physicians are taught to remain detached and objective, even in the worst of situations. But how we deal with death is at least as important as how we deal with life.

I'm not a mechanic, and I'm not a carpenter of flesh and blood. The precarious work of drilling, clipping and cutting around precious areas of memory, motor, emotional and cognitive function, and dealing with life and death decision-making has made me search for something deeper than the knife. Although he or she won't be able to point to the actual mechanism for it, a neuroscientist might see my quest in purely physiological terms, a curious product of neural processes and a particular genetic history. A rabbi or priest in turn might say I'm searching for God or the Messiah while a philosopher might explain the finite limits of explaining ourselves to ourselves. The writer and cynical humorist Tom Wolfe recently joked that the "soul" is dead: "The soul, that last refuge of values, is dead, because educated people no longer believe it exists." I couldn't disagree more. Whatever "it" is, it is alive, and no microscope, no pen—indeed, no clever theory or invention can quiet the voice calling us in the wilderness of our lives.

The New Science of Mind

Neuroscience, according to Francis Crick, is the "fifth revolution" of science in Western history. The first revolution was Copernican, the replacement of the Earth by the Sun as the center of the universe. Darwin and his theory of evolution as the origin of the species marked the second. The third revolution was Freudian, and the fourth was the discovery of the double-helix model of DNA, turning points in the understanding of the human mind and molecular biology, respectively. Up until the last decade of the twentieth century, scientists compared the human brain to a *black box*—an organ whose circuitry was unknown but whose function was understood through behavior and the expression of thought, beliefs, and emotions. The analysis of the mind has moved from the embrace of philosophers and psychologists into the arms of neuroscience. By looking at how the brain works, we can see how the mind and body function as one unit, why connections between emotions and disease exist, and how mind-body practices can not only improve your health, but literally change your mind for the better.

When I went to medical school in the 1960's, neuroscience was a nascent field. We studied the physiology of nerve cells and synapses, but the study of complex functions like learning, perception and memory had not yet extended into the realm of neurobiology. Psychology was still under the strong influence of behaviorism, what I privately considered "pseudoscience" at the time. Behaviorism was a movement that looked for patterns of behavior to explain how the mind works. The new discipline of cognitive science was just emerging. Cognitive psychology rejected the behaviorism and attempted to explain how the brain thinks and processes information from the environment. The introduction of high-tech brain scanners in the 1980's gave a huge boost to cognitive psychologists who began opening the "black box" of the brain with their new tools.

Behaviorist theories, cognitive psychology, neural science and molecular biology have united in the twenty-first century to resolve some of the questions that serious thinkers have debated for centuries. The riddle of consciousness is first on the list, and not a topic we'll discuss in-depth in this book. (Even a brain surgeon can recognize when he's in over his head). Researchers are also studying how the physical structure of the brain may contribute to exceptional talents, disabilities or pathologies. A great deal of what we know about the human brain derives from studying victims of strokes, cerebral palsy, mental illness and other diseases.

How does a three-pound, quart-sized organ packed with 1 trillion neurons and 70 trillion synaptic connections create, dream, dance or throw a winning pitch? When weighing Einstein's brain, scientists were disappointed to find no obvious differences in size or weight in comparison to the average brain. The area responsible for mathematical thought, spatial cognition, and imagery of movement, however, was remarkably different, leading neuroscientists to theorize that a lifetime of studying physics and mathematics sculpted his brain in critical ways, reinforcing what was probably an inherited potential.

Long-term brain studies have shown that the human brain is indeed more malleable than previously thought. You're born with most of the brain cells you'll ever have. But growth of the connections between brain cells determines your brain's development as an adult, a process called synaptic plasticity. A cubic millimeter of cortical tissue, the size of the "0" on your cell phone, holds about a billion synapses. Any single neuron in the brain can have between a hundred to ten thousand synaptic connections. Genes may determine your potential, but synaptic connections determine who you are.

Practice—whether it's playing golf or tennis, composing music, using a foreign language or performing yoga and brain surgery (hopefully not at the same time), literally changes the structures of the brain. Practice does not make perfect, the brain is incapable of planning the same movement each and every time. But whenever you participate in an activity that requires persistent visual or physical repetition, neural pathways grow and reorganize, forming a template for that activity. Without purpose, weaker synaptic connections wither away. Throughout a person's lifetime, synapses continually alter their strength, adding an extra layer of complexity to the brain's operations and differentiating the human brain from "hardwired" machines like the Apple computer.

When I recently asked a group of medical residents how the brain communicates with the body, everyone replied in unison, "Electrically!" The ability to perceive and interact in our rich and detailed world depends on sensory and motor impulses from the central and autonomic nervous systems, and the ligand-receptor system, your "second" nervous system. "The range of information conveyed to the brain is wider than expected, from the concentration of chemical molecules to the contractions of muscles anywhere in the body," said neurologist Eric Kandel.[99] Your nervous system interacts with every other system in your body. In the same way that all of your cells need oxygen transported by the circulatory system, all of your tissues and organs need to transmit information to and from the brain and nervous system. Understanding how the brain processes this overwhelming amount of information is crucial if we want to help people overcome or avoid pain and illnesses.

The autonomic nervous system is divided into the sympathetic and parasympathetic systems, which incorporate opposing types of nerves for involuntary body functions. The sympathetic system increases pulse and blood pressure, cools the skin and prepares the body for action. The parasympathetic system gives opposite instructions to the body. It relaxes the nerves and muscles and returns bodily functions to an even flow. The central nervous system connects all these nerves between the brain and body. It is the system which translates the intention to move a muscle into an electrical nerve impulse. All our muscular movements result from this system of communication.

Nerve impulses from the body to the brain also affect our reasoning, emotions and choices. The brain and body use the nerves in the central nervous system (CNS) and autonomic nervous system (ANS), hormones, and other chemical messengers to communicate. Most of this activity takes place at a subconscious level. Sometimes what you experience comes from activity in specialized brain regions; other times chemicals in your body change your experience. Informational molecules such as neuropeptides regulate perhaps 90 percent of our conscious and unconscious physiology. Mind and body, psychologists and neurologists now agree, aren't that different.

The molecular revolution in neuroscience changed the direction of the health and behavioral sciences, uniting neurophysiology, endocrinology and immunology with behavior, psychology and biology.[100] Like the discovery of DNA, the search for the biochemical mechanisms of emotion sparked both excitement and new discoveries about the human condition and wellness. "Physicians and academic researchers finally had the science to understand the connection between the brain and the immune system, emotions and disease," said immunologist Esther Sternberg in her book, *The Balance Within*.[101] Using the new biomolecular techniques, scientists were able to isolate and measure scores of new receptors, mapping and documenting their chemical structure. With this information, scientists in turn were able to make new external chemicals in the lab to access the cell in the same way, leading to the invention of new drug therapies for disease, depression and pain relief.

Neuroscientists know how the brain is organized anatomically and functionally, including which parts are responsible for specific functions, such as spatial memory, emotion, vision, smell, and language. Most scientists now believe that all aspects of mind, including its influence on health are explainable through a comprehensive blend of theories and facts related to all the levels of organization of the nervous system, from molecules, and cells and

Sympathetic Nervous System

FIGURE 7 The sympathetic division is principally an excitatory system that prepares the body for stress. The parasympathetic system division maintains or restores energy. Although both divisions innervate many organs and structures, the number and position of the ganglia – clusters of nerve cells where axons communicate in a synapse – are different. The activating chemicals, called neurotransmitters, and their effects are also different.

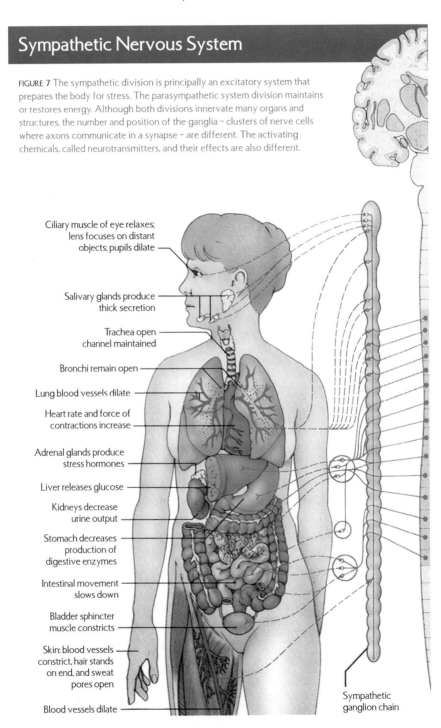

Ciliary muscle of eye relaxes; lens focuses on distant objects; pupils dilate

Salivary glands produce thick secretion

Trachea open channel maintained

Bronchi remain open

Lung blood vessels dilate

Heart rate and force of contractions increase

Adrenal glands produce stress hormones

Liver releases glucose

Kidneys decrease urine output

Stomach decreases production of digestive enzymes

Intestinal movement slows down

Bladder sphincter muscle constricts

Skin: blood vessels constrict, hair stands on end, and sweat pores open

Blood vessels dilate

Sympathetic ganglion chain

Parasympathetic Nervous System

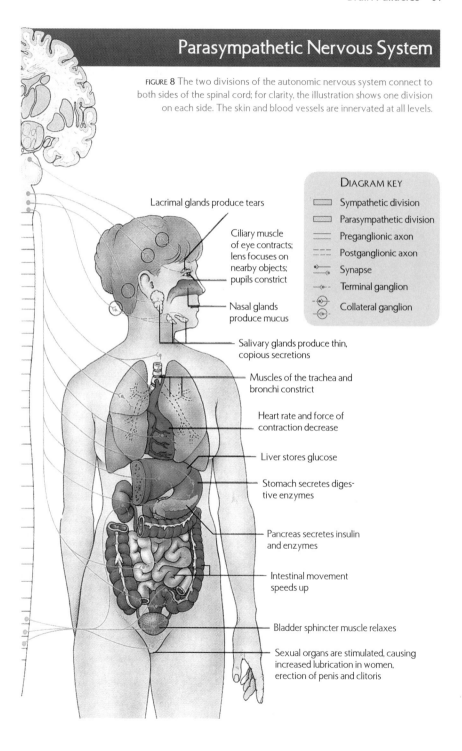

FIGURE 8 The two divisions of the autonomic nervous system connect to both sides of the spinal cord; for clarity, the illustration shows one division on each side. The skin and blood vessels are innervated at all levels.

Lacrimal glands produce tears

Ciliary muscle of eye contracts; lens focuses on nearby objects; pupils constrict

Nasal glands produce mucus

Salivary glands produce thin, copious secretions

Muscles of the trachea and bronchi constrict

Heart rate and force of contraction decrease

Liver stores glucose

Stomach secretes digestive enzymes

Pancreas secretes insulin and enzymes

Intestinal movement speeds up

Bladder sphincter muscle relaxes

Sexual organs are stimulated, causing increased lubrication in women, erection of penis and clitoris

DIAGRAM KEY

- Sympathetic division
- Parasympathetic division
- Preganglionic axon
- Postganglionic axon
- Synapse
- Terminal ganglion
- Collateral ganglion

brain circuits, to large-scale systems and physical and social environments.[102] The mind is a material product of body-wide biochemical mechanisms, and much of our behavior is determined by unconscious, automatic uptake of cues and information.

Emotions are not generated 100 percent by the brain as science had thought for decades, but also by cells themselves in blood, tissues, organs and bones. Your moods and memories are derived from complex electrochemical activity in your brain and neurochemical interactions in your body. Emotions define who we are to ourselves as well as to others. One such neurochemical of emotion is oxytocin which is also found in the heart. When the body releases oxytocin, heart rate, blood pressure and cortisol levels decrease. Humans with higher oxytocin levels are more resistant to stress and more likely to trust other people. Oxytocin levels normally rise during physical interaction of children and their mothers. Studies have shown that this rise is not observed in children that have been neglected in Eastern European orphanages and then adopted by parents in the United States.[103] These children have difficultly forming social relationships, even after being adopted into loving families, apparently because the oxytocin system has not developed to give a positive feeling about social interactions. This can change over time as the body and mind form healthier emotional pathways in the brain. Perhaps oxytocin or love is the most powerful healing emotion.

The Brain's Plasticity

A well-known example is research on London taxi drivers. To drive a traditional black cab, drivers are required to perform three years of hard training, and three-quarters of those who embark on the course drop out. After two years of study, cabbies were given brain scans by neuroscientist, Eleanor Maguire who discovered that the drivers had a larger hippocampus, a part of the brain associated with navigation compared with other people. The differences were more pronounced the longer they'd been driving. Other practices repeated over time, including Transcendental Meditation causes increases in the thickness of areas of the brain's frontal lobes associated with attention, perception and sensory processing. Brain areas associated with other skilled activities such as juggling, tennis or playing the piano or violin also increase in size with practice.

Evidence that the brain is able to change physically according to the way it is used has important implications for people who feel hardwired by genetics or suffer from brain damage or neurological disease. Your brain is a very dynamic organ which continues to grow into adulthood and beyond. Neuroplasticity is just one reason why people need to seek out places where they're surrounded by first-rate intellects, positive thinking and compassionate minds.

Young children have the largest degree of neuroplasticity. Watching violence on a regular basis not only desensitizes children to violence. If you repeatedly expose an adolescent or teen's brain to the violent images found in popular television programs, movies and video games—or if you, or a family member repeatedly displays violent behavior—you're programming your child to problem-solve through anger or violence in the real world. Adolescents who play violent video games exhibit changes in brain physiology that may underlie more aggressive behaviors that may be not able to control, according to research from Indiana University medical school.[104]

Another common fallacy is that the brain has isolated areas of "reason" or "emotion." No fixed hierarchy exists in the brain. Any given mental task involves a web of circuits that interact with informational substances. Classical views on how the brain operates divided sensing from understanding and assigned each faculty (such as memory) a separate seat in the cortex. Neurologist Paul MacLean's triune brain theory described the human cerebrum in three layers, representing different stages of evolution. At the bottom is the brain stem or primitive brain, which drives the basic needs of life (blood pressure, body temperature and other autonomic functions). Grafted on top of the brain stem are the limbic system or the "seat of emotions;" and the neocortex, the "seat of the intellect." MacLean theorized that neocortex dominated the more primitive levels of the brain. With the advent of modern technologies, we have new information about how the mind works.

Profound division of labor or functional specialization occurs in several areas of the brain previously thought to be sole areas of one faculty. Specialized areas connect with one another, either directly or through other areas. Your brain has no decision-making center—it's an associative network with competing subsystems or specialized "modules." Brain systems work in tandem via biochemical and nerve connections in the body. A specialized region in the frontal lobes related to making personal and social decisions works in concert with deeper brain centers that store emotional memories.[105] What you're doing, thinking or feeling depends on the activity of these networked modules.[106]

When we experience certain events in our mind or our environment, a stimulus triggers a component of the brain that leads to changes in our bodies and vice-versa. For instance, a perceived threat might lead to changes in facial expression, sweat glands, and breathing and heart rate. The brain is only a small part of a broader self. According to Daniel Siegel, the author of *The Developing Mind*:

> It is crucial in understanding the mind and its development
> that we embrace the exciting findings from brain science
> while exploring the reality that brain and mind are *not* the
> same. Since energy and information can flow beyond the
> boundaries of the skin-defined self, mind is a process that is
> beyond merely brain anatomy and biology.[107]

Circuit firing from the frontal cortex can go deeply down into the body. The mind is organized like the Internet—you can readily access it by the ear, the hand or any other place in the body. We perceive the world through our senses. The inward movie of thought, sight and sound and touch is bound into the illusion of self. "To live is so startling it leaves little time for anything else," said Emily Dickinson. New molecular and pharmaceutical tools have made it possible to map the active network that exists between the brain's anatomy and circuitry and the body's sense organs—the nose, eyes, ears, mouth and tongue, and the skin. Physiological responses become physical sensations that we associate with emotions. Emotions in turn affect behavior and choices. These are called altered states of consciousness, different states of mind, emotions, memories or postures.

Another popular myth is that we only use 10 percent of our brain. Functional brain scans showing conscious human subjects thinking or performing a task reveal lots of areas of the brain lighting up. Your mind is an associative network. Perception and comprehension occur simultaneously:

> It's no longer possible to divide the process of seeing from
> that of understanding, as neurologists once imagined, nor is
> it possible to separate the acquisition of visual knowledge
> form consciousness. Indeed, consciousness is a property of

the complex neural apparatus that the brain has developed to acquire knowledge.[108]

We also think of the mind as consciousness or the self. The illusion of the self—the individual with free will—is actually a series of neural circuits and chemical messengers throughout the body that work in parallel to create a unified consciousness. As William James said a century ago, "Consciousness is not a thing but a process."[109] No single area of the body synthesizes all the incoming information—sensory experience and emotions are intertwined throughout the body. What you experience as "self" is the result of simultaneous maneuvers of mind and body.

The hippocampus, the area of the brain associated with memory is linked through nerve pathways to sensory parts of the brain and to the frontal lobe which filters thoughts and emotions. That's why the odor of autumn leaves reminds me of my first day of school, or the smell of matzo ball soup on the stove reminds me of my mother. The nose has roughly 1,000 different odor receptors, yet we can perceive no less than 10,000 smells. Each characteristic scent is a mix of odorant molecules that activates a combination of different sensors, types of receptor cells that send their signal via the olfactory bulb to the brain's cortex. Linda B. Buck and Richard Axel won a Nobel Prize for mapping how signals from those receptors are arranged in higher regions of the brain to yield diverse odor perceptions. Scientists are studying the neural processes that correlate with a particular conscious experience like the perception of smell or vision to understand how the brain and body decipher the world around us. Social neuroscientists expands the unit of analysis to two brains—interactions that affect the neurology of two people.

How Social Interaction Heals

"Social neurobiology" is an emerging scientific field that combines neuroscience with social psychology to explore the neurobiological mechanisms of social interactions. One of the most important areas of study involves mapping psychological situations, such as moral dilemmas, onto neurobiology. Social neuroscientists discovered that empathy involves a class of nerve cells in the brain that allows people to mimic motor actions, emotions, and social behaviors. These nerve cells, called "mirror neurons," follow the emotional current, actions and even the intentions of the person we are with, and replicate these states in the same areas of the brain as the other person. Mirror neurons connect us automatically with another person or in a community such as a family, school, corporation, church or even the Internet. Social neuroscientists claim mirror neurons may explain character traits or dispositions that equip people for success with interpersonal relationships, including empathy, kindness, faith, generosity, trust and forgiveness.

Gregory L. Fricchione, M.D., an associate professor of psychiatry at Harvard Medical School, attributed mirror neurons to the reflex actions of a father who saved a young man from an oncoming subway train in New York. He explained that when the man saw the stranger fall onto the tracks, his thalamus, which absorbs sensory information, registered the fall, and sent the information to other parts of the brain for processing. The amygdala, the part of the brain that mediates fear responses, sent sensory information to the motor cortex for emotional processing. The anterior cingulate, a key decision-making area, kicked in, helping trigger a decision about how to act.

The Neurobiology of Empathy

The human brain has multiple mirror neuron systems that specialize in performing and understanding not just the movement of others but their intentions and the social and emotional meaning of their behavior. Human relationships shape your brain's neural connections. According to Daniel Goleman in *Social Intelligence*, "Mirror neurons offer a neural mechanism that explains emotional contagion, the tendency of one person to catch the feelings of another, particularly if strongly expressed."[110] Neuroscientists and psychologists think that mirror neurons allow us to grasp the minds of others through intuition, not by thinking.

Circuits in your brain, which neuroscientists do not yet entirely understand, inhibit you from moving while you simulate an action with mirror neurons. You understand the action because you have in your brain a template for that action based on your own movements. Neuroscientist Giacomo Rizzolatti gave these examples in a recent *New York Times* article:

If you see me choke up in emotional distress, mirror neurons in your brain simulate my distress. You automatically have empathy for me. You know how I feel because you literally feel what I am feeling …When you see a spider crawl up someone's leg, you feel a creepy sensation because your mirror neurons are firing.[111]

This intuitive link may also account for empathy, which research finds depend in part on rapid-fire brain processing of people's posture, voice and behavior. Mirror neurons fire when you see or hear an action and when you carry out the same action on your own. Researchers at UCLA found that cells in the human anterior cingulate, which normally fire when you poke the patient with a needle, will also fire when the patient watches another patient being poked. The mirror neurons, it would seem, dissolve the barrier between self and others.

Simply imagining that you're doing something leaves a mark on the brain as well. Artists, writers, professional athletes and coaches have used mental practice and imagery to exploit the brain's mirror properties for years. Observation also improves muscle performance via mirror neurons—muscle-memory. In Pavlov's case, the dogs associated the sound of a bell with the sight of food and learned to salivate merely at the sound of the bell. A century later, molecular biologists have the tools to look for biochemical salivations in neurons that change when they associate these stimuli. Geneticist Tim Tully's experiment on "photographic memory" in fruit flies was the first demonstration of genetically enhanced memory in history. Tully, who investigates the genetic basis of memory, believes neurons are built to reconfigure or retune themselves on the basis of associative stimuli in the environment. He encourages physical exercise to promote neuronal survival and reduce the damaging effects (cell death) of stress. By combining strong positive thoughts, verbal affirmations and deep breathing with movement, the brain and body can generate healing biochemicals.

CHAPTER 6

The Neurobiology of Stress

Future shock [is] the shattering stress and disorientation that we induce in individuals by subjecting them to too much change in too short a time.

– Alvin Toffler

Less than a century ago, the word "stress" wasn't a part of the American lexicon. Engineers working on the Brooklyn Bridge in Lower Manhattan understood the technical term as "mechanical forces acting on physical structures." According to linguist, author and pundit William Safire, stress, the noun, is a shortening of distress, rooted in the Latin distringere, "to hinder, molest." Stress, the verb, has another root as well: the Latin stringere, "to draw tight, press together," which is related to strain. Today stress has come to take its meaning from the verb: "pressure: whether through direct force, tension exerted on a person or thing." Pressure, tension and stress, which are synonymous in general use, lead to anxiety and strain. The vogue term was presaged by John Locke circa 1698: "Though the faculties of the mind are improved by exercise, yet they must not be put to a stress beyond their strength."

Stress is the inability to cope with a *perceived* (real or imagined) threat to one's mental, physical, emotional, and spiritual well-being, which results in a series of physiological responses and adaptations.[113] Internal stressors can also be physical (infections, inflammation) or psychological. External stressors include adverse physical conditions (such as pain or hot or cold temperatures) or stressful psychological environments. Medically speaking, stress is the non-specific response of the body to any demand. The presence of stress causes physical, measurable changes, such as an increase in pulse, respiration and heart rate. Virtually all systems—cardiovascular, pulmonary, digestive, endocrine, immune and nervous—act to meet the perceived danger. Stress has replaced infectious agents of disease as the number one health evil facing Western culture.

In the 1920s, physiologist Walter Cannon first used the term "stress" to describe the body's response to unpleasant conditions, named the "fight or flight response." Cannon described in his classic, *The Wisdom of the Body* that the body had automatic control over functions such as temperature control, digestion and heart rate. A single nerve, called the vagus, that exits at the back of the brain and continues down the body via the spinal cord and nerve branches, can send signals to the body's organs, including the pupils of the eyes, the salivary glands, the heart, the bronchi of the lungs, the stomach, the intestines, the bladder, the sex organs and the adrenal glands. When Cannon stimulated the vagus nerve through electrodes implanted in the brain's hypothalamus just above the pituitary gland, he discovered that there were physiological changes in all of these organs consistent with the body's response to an emergency. Blood, for example, was re-routed from the internal organs of digestion to the muscles. An increase of adrenaline stimulated the heart and caused the liver to release extra sugar for instant energy.

Acute stress stimulates the sympathetic adrenal system and an outpouring of adrenalin-like hormones that prepare the body for "fight or flight." Pupils dilate, blood pressure and heart rate rise and blood flow to the brain increases, resulting in improved vision and other cerebral functions. Glycogen stores in the liver rapidly break down into glucose to provide immediate energy. Blood shunts from the gut to the muscles of the arms and legs so that we can run faster. Blood also clots more rapidly to diminish loss from any hemorrhage. In short, a host of potentially life-saving physiological and chemical events occur under the body's stress response.

Hans Selye, a charismatic and influential neuroendocrinologist popularized the notion that stress (and the emotional or physical reaction to it) can make people sick. Building on Cannon's model of the "fight or flight" response to a generalized notion of stress, Selye proposed that over time, harsh environments (including the stress of modern living) can cause increasing levels of physical stress eventually resulting in physical syndromes, exhaustion and even death. In his landmark study published in 1950, *The Physiology and Pathology of Exposure to Stress*, Selye theorized that poor adaptation to stress was the basis of most illnesses and disease. His theories permeated medical thinking and influenced medical research for twenty years, replacing psychoanalytically-based psychosomatic theories.

About 10 years later, physicist Elmer Green developed biofeedback techniques in which patients learned to control unconscious processes. Under his care, patients watched monitoring devices that tracked things like heart rate or blood pressure. By observing how their different actions affect data readouts, patients could start to voluntarily regulate certain body functions such as blood pressure. Green's experience led him to state:

> Every change in the physiological state is accompanied by an
> appropriate change in the mental emotional state, conscious
> or unconscious, and conversely, every change in the
> emotional state, conscious or unconscious, is accompanied by
> an appropriate change in the physiological state.[113]

Herbert Benson found that under most circumstances, once the acute threat has passed, the response becomes inactivated and levels of stress hormones return to normal, a condition called the *relaxation response*. The problem is that contemporary life poses on-going stressful situations that are not short-lived and the urge to act (to fight or to flee) must be suppressed or the fight-or-flight response becomes perpetual.

The physiology of stress and the fight-or-flight response has been studied and publicized more than any other neurochemical process. The body's stress response activates the brain's hypothalamus and pituitary glands, which regulate hormones, particularly the stress hormone cortisol that regulates immune functioning, blood pressure, insulin and proper glucose metabolism. While small increases in cortisol improve performance, long-term (chronic) exposure to stress hormones can cause atrophy of the brain's hippocampus, leading to memory impairment. To make matters worse, we pour adrenalin into our bodies with cans of popular energy drinks; double-shot, three-pump, grandé café lattes; or popular movies and television shows—all of which causes our body and mind to endure even more stress. High cortisol levels also increase food intake and contribute to central body fat, a condition my colleagues in cardiology refer to as "toxic fat." Abdominal fat, insulin resistance or glucose intolerance, high blood pressure, inflammation and bad cholesterol are known to increase the progression of heart disease.

Prolonged stress also can be hazardous to brain function, hormone production, immune responses, and other processes.[114] Stress-related disorders and diseases brought on or worsened by psychological stress commonly involve the autonomic nervous system, which controls the body's internal organs, including the heart, lungs and brain.

Chronically stressed individuals have increased levels of the stress hormone cortisol, which slows the delivery of immune cells and molecules to injury sites. In turn, this slows the start of the healing process. In 2004, a twenty-year long study proved that the longer the duration of a stressor, the greater the disruption of pro-inflammatory cytokines which in turn may increase susceptibility to viruses that cause the common cold.[115] The study also showed that social relationships may influence wellness and recovery from disease. Social isolation such as loneliness raised blood pressure. Alzheimer's caregivers were more likely to have severe colds. Bereavement and unemployment lowered lymphocyte counts up to two months after the initial stressor. Couples going through a divorce have depressed T and NK cells, immune cells that strengthen resistance to infection. And research on wound healing suggests that marital stress delays healing and increases the body's production of pro-inflammatory cytokines that can accelerate a range of age-related diseases, such as heart disease.[116] Depressing life events, such as divorce or the death of a loved one, can even create enough stress to interfere with the heart's pump, causing "broken-heart syndrome," a temporary heart failure that can lead to death if not treated.

People are more susceptible to illness when under stress, including young students who create fewer antibodies to the flu vaccine around exam time. When the reasons for patients' visits to physicians are examined, between 60-90 percent of visits are related to stress and other psychosocial factors.[117] In my own practice, I've discovered that a ten-minute "stress survey" is an important diagnostic tool. Physicians need to integrate stress evaluations into standard history-taking and examinations.

American's advanced technical society is responsible for much of the information overload that causes stress, and generalized anxiety will affect all adults to some degree at different points in their life. The constant influx of information from mass communication systems such as blogging, video-teleconferencing, mobile phones, e-mail, snail mail, text messaging, instant messaging, landlines, advertisements, telemarketers and voicemail and the information output from the Internet, newspapers, magazines, newsletters, billboards, satellite television and radio causes a certain degree of information angst in everyone. Consider life in America only 100 years ago: Only 8 percent of homes had a telephone; 8,000 cars were on the road; the speed limit was 10 MPH; and there were only 144 miles of paved roads. Today the information highway connects people across the planet, opening the door not just to our neighboring country's cultural nuances, but the complex socioeconomic realities of second and third world countries which seemed remote but the impact of 9/11 will forever remind us that the world is in our backyard. Our hearts and minds haven't caught up with technology's great lurch forward.

Stress levels rise for different reasons and in different seasons, around national holidays and periods of economic instability and recession. Post 9/11, a nationwide survey published in the *NEJM* found that 90 percent of American adults experienced a stress-related symptom. Following an economic recession, the Department of Health, Education, and Infectious Disease Center in Atlanta revealed nationwide increases in ulcers, heart attacks, impotency, weight loss and depression. You may want to consider heading to the tanning booth the next time you're feeling in a funk. Light therapy and even tanning booths have been shown to raise serotonin levels in the organ of the skin, and can help people who suffer from seasonal affective disorder.

Job stress is one of the most universal and chronic kinds of stress. Technically, job stress is "lack of harmony between the individual and his or her work environment." Employment losses are often followed by an increase in heart attacks, hypertension, ulcers and other pain-related illnesses and even death. Factory work and jet lag are known to create discordance between natural body rhythms and daily activities, resulting in disordered sleep patterns, mood disorders and other medical problems. In factory work, the risk of accidental injury is significantly increased during the night shift. Perhaps more disturbing is a recent report that destruction of the brain's master clock rendered mice more susceptible to experimentally induced cancers.[118]

The American idolization of youth in media such as films and television programs and marketing or advertisements also creates a kind of unconscious stress. In contrast to many Eastern countries such as China and Japan, older Americans are unsupported by family members who are often scattered all over the country or overwhelmed with their immediate responsibilities. Foreigners often criticize Americans for consigning the aged disabled to nursing homes or senior-citizen communities, a concept that doesn't exist in most countries.

Time-pressured activity is another common cause of stress. The Earth moves on a 24-hour cycle and so do we. Our body clocks synchronize us to our environment, and even to the seasons' changing day lengths. For this we can thank circadian rhythms, temporal programs of around 24 hours found in virtually all living things. Their most obvious signature is our sleep–wake cycles. But research on a wide range of organisms is revealing many clocks, working at levels from the cellular to the whole-animal.

The body's main circadian pacemaker is found deep within the brain's hypothalamus which receives direct input from the retina. A recently discovered class of photoreceptors not involved in image generation, contains a light-sensitive pigment. Even blind people lacking functional vision can respond to light signals with the retina's photoreceptors. The brain's "master clock" orchestrates a wide range of neural and hormonal signals, which drive a multitude of cyclical responses around the body, making routine sleep a critical component of rejuvenation and wellness.

Adding to stress is the fact that organized religion has waned drastically in modern Western society, leaving people stranded in a materialistic society with no clear belief system. A general feeling of incompleteness or spiritual vacuum haunts many people today, promoting a degree of confusion in values. The popular spiritual debate between scientists and people of faith may make some people feel like they have to choose sides: the cold, fact-filled universe of biological evolution or the supernatural world of miracles and faith. St. Augustine, one of the greatest Western thinkers warns against a narrow perspective of the creation story in Genesis. In my opinion, the human spirit requires neither religion nor reliance on miracles; the inherent quality or particularity to the human condition is the result of wondrous adaptive biological mechanisms that protect, sustain and perpetuate our existence.

Stress and High Blood Pressure

High blood pressure often occurs earlier in life, is more severe and has more complications in African-American men and women. And yet, blacks are less likely to seek treatment until their blood pressure has been high for so long that vital organs have already started to suffer damage. Denial is often a component in seeking treatment, but so are lack of access to medical care; misdiagnosis; lack of awareness about inexpensive preventative self-care; and dismissive doctors. Women, especially, have no feeling of empowerment when it comes to their own health care. And for good reason—several studies have shown that when it comes to women, physicians don't listen as well, preventative medications aren't prescribed as much, diagnostic tests aren't as accurate, and women's symptoms are harder to recognize.[119]

A terrible case example took place in 2006 when forty-nine year old Beatrice arrived at an emergency room in Ohio complaining of nausea, shortness of breath and chest pains. A nurse saw her briefly and told her to wait. Her daughter twice told the hospital staff that her mother needed immediate care. But two hours later, when Beatrice's name was finally called, the staff found her slumped in a chair, already dead. Patients suffering from an apparent heart attack must be put on cardiac monitoring immediately within 10 minutes of their arrival. The coroner said in Beatrice's case, none of that happened. A coroner's jury investigating the case ruled Beatrice's death a homicide, opening the door for criminal prosecution.

Critical delays in the detection, accurate diagnosis and proper treatment of vascular diseases that threaten women's lives. The racial disparity in survival for disease and illness is multi-factorial, and the more we learn about the origins, both genetic and environmental, the more capable doctors will be in developing more tailored screening, preventive and therapeutic strategies for high-risk patients in the future. The pioneering neurosurgeon Harvey Cushing said almost a century ago, "A physician must consider more than a diseased organ, more than the whole person; the physician must view the person in his or her world."

African-Americans on average have *double* the rate of hypertension in comparison to whites.[120] Among the reasons for such disparities between white and blacks, we might consider the stress experienced by African-Americans, striving to overcome negative stereotypes and prove themselves against a backdrop of racism and inequality about which they are acutely aware. Our reactions to others have far-reaching biological impacts, triggering a cascade of destructive or positive internal chemicals. Under stress, the body shuts down resources from the endocrine and immune systems and releases hormones that fuel the body to act. These hormones also trigger inflammatory mechanisms known to influence the development of diabetes and hypertension. The elevation of inflammation is likely a key reason why metabolic syndrome leads to accelerated coronary disease risk in women.[121]

Acute Manifestations of Stress

Everyone has a story related to stress. My most notable one is about Scott, then a globe-trotting, Google-clicking, dot.com executive. Scott headed the nuts and bolts of developing an online service in China, which was not an easy feat when you consider Beijing's obsession to control free speech over an Internet spanning half-a-billion users. He had been flying back and forth to Asia to carve-out the terms of a multi-million dollar deal with China's largest PC manufacturer. Two weeks spent in the purple pollution haze of Beijing would send most people to the hospital, but Scott went about his business and rushed home in time for a wedding. Upon arriving stateside after the fourteen-hour flight, his back began to itch. When he took off his shirt and asked his wife to look at the rash with a copy of the consumer edition of the *Merck Manual* in hand, she diagnosed him with shingles. Shingles is caused by the varicella-zoster virus, the same virus that causes chickenpox. After you've had chickenpox, the virus lies dormant in your nerves. Years later, the virus may reactivate under stress.

A week later, Scott woke up with a fever, stiff neck and the worst headache of his life. His wife left a bridal shower to take him to the Emergency Room, where he was evaluated for meningitis, an infection and inflammation of the membranes (meninges) and cerebrospinal fluid surrounding your brain and spinal cord. Meningitis is a rare complication of shingles. When I arrived at the hospital, Scott laid in the dark on a gurney with a bucket beside his head. He was overcome by pain so severe that he vomited continuously, making a spinal tap to confirm the diagnosis "difficult." After testing positive for viral meningitis (bacterial meningitis can progress to widespread infection of the nervous system, leading to shock and death within days), I ordered an IV with the anti-viral medication, Val acyclovir and morphine. Complications of meningitis include permanent hearing loss, blindness, loss of speech and brain damage leading to paralysis or even death.

Shingles is rare for people under 50 years old. You're more susceptible to shingles if you have cancer or a weakened immune system. I asked Scott's wife, a thin woman with a tall forehead and large blue eyes, if he was under a lot of stress. She told me that day in and day out for months Scott bowed to business demands in more ways than one. He was making the fourteen-hour flight from Washington, DC to Beijing so often that he earned the prestigious 1K status in mileage awards. His cell phone, computer and Blackberry buzzed late in the evening and early in the morning because of the twelve-hour time difference in business hours. She said she could often hear Scott raising his voice and repeating himself on nightly conference calls in their library, irritated with translators who often botched key terms in English, resulting in confusion and delays.

After a week in the hospital and several weeks of in-home nursing care, Scott fully recovered. Because I was concerned that he may have brushed up against a rare disease from a region famous for breeding deadly pandemics, I referred him to an "international" epidemiologist for a battery of tests. His blood work was 100 percent normal, implying that his shingles had been triggered by stress.

As Scott's story illustrates, stress is your body's perception of a physical or psychological threat and being ill prepared for it. The "fight-or-flight" response results in your body's release of stress hormones—adrenaline or noradrenalin. The short-term impact of stress includes increased metabolic, heart and breathing rates. The long-term, chronic impact can be a weakened immune system, cardiac arrhythmias, hypertension, abdominal cramping and diarrhea, and muscle tension. Inflammatory diseases that are shown to be associated with an abrupt stress response are rheumatoid arthritis, Lupus, dermatitis and asthma.

Healing Stress-related Illness

Learned attitudes through cultural, religious and family experiences strongly influence the way people adapt to stress. Everyone has a highly complex set of beliefs and attitudes. Each one of us sees things, including stress, in a totally different way.

Current pharmaceutical and surgical approaches cannot adequately treat stress-related illness. Holistic mind-body approaches, including nutrition, exercise, and motivating patients to change their belief structures, can help people better cope with the endemic stress of our culture. Most adults operate on a level of necessary and tolerable stress to improve performance. However, excessive, long-term stress reaction can lead to illness and disease or non-physical pain syndromes. Our physiology wasn't created or didn't evolve fast enough to cope with the burden of the kind of repeated stress and anxiety prevalent today. Emotions affect which details we remember. And things that trigger strong emotional responses—like stressful car accidents or violent images on television—are recalled more readily according to renowned psychologist, Kevin Ochsner.

Ochsner's research at Columbia University examines the psychological and neural processes involved in extracting emotional and cognitive meaning from the world. His research interests include the psychological and neural processes involved in emotion, pain and selfhood using neuroscience methods such as fMRI and the study of brain lesion populations. Perhaps one of the most valuable findings of his research is that when we're experiencing something disturbing, our brain records more details than if we were experiencing something relaxing or pleasurable.

Over a century ago, Freud proposed that people can exclude unwanted memories from awareness, a process called "repression." It was unknown, however, how repression occurs in the brain. Oschner's team used fMRI to identify the neural systems involved in keeping unwanted memories out of awareness. Controlling unwanted memories was associated with increased prefrontal activation, reduced activation of the hippocampus, and impaired retention of those memories, confirming the existence of an active forgetting process and establishing a neurobiological model for guiding inquiry into motivated forgetting. This provides a psychological model for the voluntary form of repression (suppression) proposed by Freud.

One theory for stress-related illness is that it results from repression of stress or stress-related memories. That is, part of our brain wants to react while another part tries to restrain, which results in tension. The thinking part of your brain—the prefrontal lobes located in the front part of your brain—doesn't allow you to scream out. (Think of Edvard Munch's painting, *The Scream*). The amygdala would have us screaming and jumping from tree to tree. A lot of your negative thoughts and emotions about stress are stored in the subconscious, the unconscious part of your mind where memories, feelings or thoughts influence your behavior without your awareness. This is the key when dealing with stress-related illnesses. According to John Sarno, M.D.:

Your brain tries to shove any threatening emotions into your unconscious so you don't have to become aware of them. When the feelings aren't all that intense or threatening, your brain manages to keep them repressed. However, when the emotions are particularly strong, it's harder to keep them tucked away, so your brain needs to create a distraction. It creates real physiological changes in your body, which in turn create real symptoms. These symptoms are painful or distressing enough to take your attention away from the threatening, unacceptable feelings.[122]

Prolonged stress and the conditioned impulse to restrain negative emotions like anger or frustration can produce incremental changes in the brain and immune system over many years. Emotional tension related to repression of negative memories, emotion and stress contributes to the majority of pain-related, psychogenic illness—the symptoms become a distraction from the original stimulus.

Stress-provoking images, sounds and situations can cause people (especially children) to overproduce stress hormones, including the adrenal hormone cortisol, which is responsible for much of the physical damage caused by long-term stress. Chronic elevations of stress hormones contribute to a host of illnesses, including asthma, gastric ulcers and cardiovascular disease. Children who are shy or inhibited in unfamiliar situations have been shown to suffer from multiple allergic disorders. Some of the most disturbing research on stress is showing that persistent elevations of cortisol increases the vulnerability of neurons in the hippocampus to damage by other substances; this brain region influences motivation, memory and emotion.

The body's stress response operates autonomously but can be conditioned through the techniques we discuss in Part IV. To better understand the mechanics of stress, you'll need to learn a few simple insights about the brain's multitasking functionality and the body's process of activating the stress response.

Mapping Stress

Stress starts with a perceived threat, the root of all fear, which causes the body's fight-or-flight response. The adrenal glands send adrenalin, noradrenalin and cortisol into the bloodstream, quickening the heartbeat and raising blood pressure. The sympathetic nervous system helps redirect blood to the muscles, constricting arteries and reducing blood flow to the internal organs. Fat cells are released into the bloodstream for quick energy, which are not all reabsorbed. The release of stress hormones makes blood platelets stickier, which might lead to the accumulation of plaque. This process occurs over and over in people who are easily stressed. But in the chronically angry, the damage is amplified because the response itself is sharper.

Using a "hostility questionnaire" and angiograms, researchers have found that most hostile men have more severe arteriosclerosis. Researchers at the University of Miami recently found that HIV-positive people who took part in stress management workshops showed improved endocrine and immune functions.

Specific brain and body regions process fear, emotions, and the physiological stress response. The brain is divided into the cerebrum, diencephalons, brain stem, and cerebellum. Three interconnection brain regions regulate fear: the prefrontal cortex, the amygdala, and the hypothalamus.

The frontal lobes of the cerebrum, including the prefrontal cortex, make up 60 percent of the brain hemispheres and extend from the back of the eyes to the middle of the ears. The prefrontal cortex interprets sensory stimuli and evaluates potential danger. The frontal lobes are the "executive planning center" of the brain, enabling us to calculate, coordinate, and plan. When trauma or disease affects the frontal lobes we may become apathetic, lethargic and unable to start or complete new tasks. Some of us may become uninhibited and start gambling impulsively and recklessly, becoming obsessed sexually and picking fights.

The second region involved in fear and aggression is the amygdala, almond-shaped regions in the limbic system. Limbic means border. The limbic system borders the cortex (upper part of the brain) and the subcortex (lower part of the brain). The amygdala performs a primary role in the processing and memory of emotional reactions. Infants are born with well-developed amygdala, which is why a baby cries when picked up by an unfamiliar person or taken to an unfamiliar place. Fear is a primitive survival tactic. Autistics have a highly-reduced amygdala; they are unable to process several emotions, including the comprehension of fear or aggression in people's faces or behavioral expressions. The lack of inhibition and stimulus-seeking

The Brain's Limbic System

FIGURE 9 The components of this ring-shaped system play a complex and important role in the expression of instincts, drives, and emotions. They mediate the effects of moods on external behavior and influence internal changes in bodily function and their appropriate expression. The association of feelings with sensations, such as smell and sight, and the formation of memories are also influenced by the limbic system.

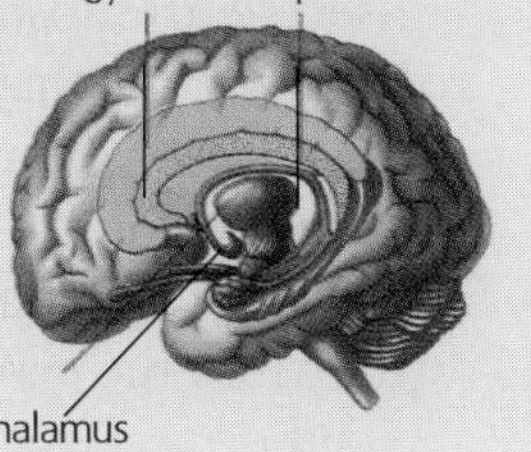

Cingulate gyrus   Corpus callosum

Thalamus

LOCATION OF THE LIMBIC SYSTEM

The limbic system encircles the top of the brain stem and forms a border (the meaning of "limbic") linking cortical and midbrain areas with lower centers that control automatic, internal body functions.

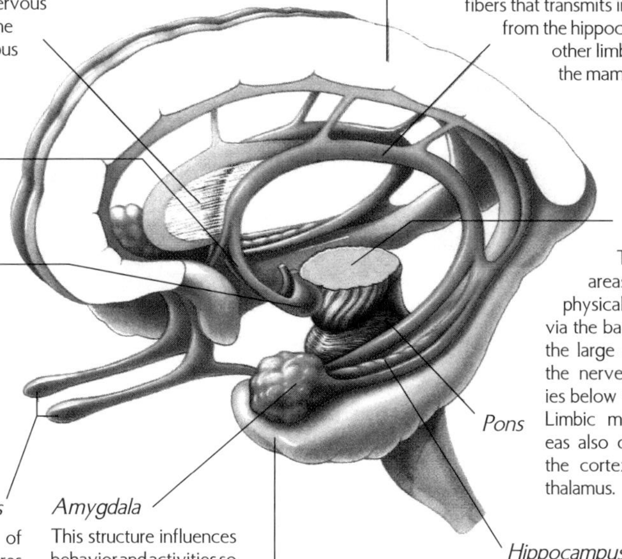

Cingulate gyrus
This area, together with the parahippocampal gyrus and the olfactory bulbs, comprises the limbic cortex, which modifies behavior and emotions.

Septum pellucidum
A thin sheet of nervous tissue connects the fornix to the corpus callosum.

Fornix
The fornix is a pathway of nerve fibers that transmits information from the hippocampus and other limbic areas to the mamillary body.

Column of fornix

Midbrain
The limbic areas influence physical activity via the basal ganglia, the large clusters of the nerve cell bodies below the cortex. Limbic midbrain areas also connect to the cortex and the thalamus.

Mamillary body
This tiny nucleus acts as a relay station, transmitting information to and from the fornix and the thalamus.

Pons

Olfactory bulbs
The connection of these structures with the limbic system helps explain why the sense of smell evokes long forgotten memories and emotions.

Amygdala
This structure influences behavior and activities so that they are appropriate for meeting the body's internal needs. These include feeding, sexual interest, and emotional reactions such as anger.

Parahippocampal gyrus
With other structures, this area helps modify the expression of emotions such as rage and fright.

Hippocampus
This curved band of gray matter is involved with learning and memory, the recognition of novelty, and the recollection of spatial relationships.

behavior associated with Attention-Deficit Hyperactivity Disorder also may be due to disrupted connections between the amygdala and frontal cortex. The amygdala is your key to intuition.

Neuroscientists think that the amygdala reacts without input from the thinking part of the brain. "An emotional reaction like fear can more easily gain control over the cortex and influence cortical processes than the cortex can gain control over the amygdala."[123] During a stressful event, the amygdala sends impulses to the hypothalamus for activation of the sympathetic nervous system and other important brain regions for increased reflexes, facial expressions and activation of dopamine and adrenaline hormones.

Sometimes emotions can be triggered without the cortex knowing exactly what's going on. Neuroscientists refer to these emotional explosions as "neural hijackings."[124] A key emotional area deep in the center of the brain, once again the amygdala, proclaims an emergency, recruiting the rest of the mind and body to act. The hijacking occurs in an instant, overriding the thinking or judging part of the brain, the neocortex. Today, one in 20 Americans may be susceptible to repeated, uncontrollable emotional outbursts in which they lash out in physical abuse, road rage or other unjustifiably violent actions.[125] Scientists at Harvard and the University of Chicago say that neural hijackings are on the rise, and substance abuse is a typically a complicating factor. In some people with mental disorders, this may be especially strong, so their emotions are being triggered in ways that prevent them from having insight into what they are doing.

Fear follows two simultaneous paths in the brain: 1) the *unconscious*, intuitive recognition of danger flashes in the amygdala, and 2) the *conscious* executive decision-making that takes place in the prefrontal cortex.[126] The amygdala also performs primary roles in the formation and storage of detailed-memories associated with emotional events. Military members in the Middle East have to be alert for surprise attacks anyplace, anytime. The emotional and psychological conditioning can have lasting effects. For example, after the Afghan war, one of my friends said that the long, drooping clusters of Spanish moss on the Live Oak trees in his backyard became ominous; they were ideal perches with camouflage for snipers. He removed the long, grayish-green filaments of moss. Studies on post-traumatic stress disorder connect an overabundance of fear memories in the amygdala with an inability to consciously discriminate danger from harmless phenomena.

The centrally-located diencephalons in the brain include the thalamus, hypothalamus and epithalamus. The thalamus is about 80 percent of the diencephalons, and serves as a critical relay station for sensory impulses, except for the sense of smell. The thalamus receives visual information from the eyes, auditory information from the ears, and sensory information from the body. It processes and analyzes this information and then relays it for further processing. The hypothalamus is a small region below the thalamus.

The main function of the hypothalamus is homeostasis, or maintaining the body's status quo. Factors such as blood pressure, body temperature, fluid and electrolyte balance, and body weight are held to a precise value called the set-point. Although this set-point can migrate over time, from day to day it is remarkably fixed. Many doctors still believe the hypothalamus is the chief center governing the emotional aspect of human life. More current research supports the interaction of the brain's structures, neuropeptides, hormones and neurotransmitters to create the chemical, electrical and physiologic state of the living organism. There can be differences of opinion about this, but most neurologists and neurosurgeons, as well as the rest of the medical community, still does not appreciate the great influence of neuropeptides on the body.

A substantial portion of human cellular machinery is dedicated to maintaining homeostasis. In response to stress signals from the amygdala, the hypothalamus secretes corticotrophin-releasing hormone (CRH). This is a key hormone shared by the central nervous system and immune system, uniting the stress and immune responses. CRH triggers the pituitary gland to secrete adrenocorticotropic hormone (ACTH), which in turn spurs the adrenal gland to produce cortisol.

Cortisol is a steroid hormone that helps you meet the demands of stress. It's also a potent anti-inflammatory agent, playing a critical role in preventing the immune system from damaging tissues. Cortisol is essential, so its levels in the blood are closely controlled. When cortisol levels rise, ACTH levels normally fall. When cortisol levels fall, ACTH levels normally rise. The body's response to cortisol is to increase blood pressure and to decrease the pulse rate. Other internal changes include a decrease in the number of white blood cells and an increase in the rate that amino acids (protein) change into sugar (glucose). CRH and cortisol are two important keys to the mind-body connection.

CRH-secreting neurons of the hypothalamus regulate the autonomic nervous center (ANS), as well as the "locus ceruleus," an area of the brain stem involved in arousal, fear and enhanced vigilance. The ANS is an entire little brain unto itself; its name comes from "autonomous," and it runs bodily functions without our awareness or control, although we can consciously alter it through techniques such as focus, meditation and breathing exercises. The ANS includes two systems that often oppose each other: the sympathetic and parasympathetic systems.

The parasympathetic system has many specific functions, including slowing the heart, constricting the pupils, stimulating the gut and salivary glands, and other responses that are not a priority when threatened by danger. The body's parasympathetic or the "relaxation response" can be solicited through soothing music, laughter, nature and other inexpensive, non-pharmaceutical techniques such as breathing deeply. The sympathetic system evokes responses characteristic of the "fight-or-flight" response when pupils dilate, muscles tense, heart rate increases, and the digestive system is put on hold. It also stimulates immune organs, such as the spleen. Our knowledge about how the brain processes emotion has been gleaned through the study of the stress response. We'll give you the "play-by-play" of a familiar scene to provide a glimpse into your internal disaster-response team.

You're driving and talking on your cell phone. The right parietal lobes of your brain help judge spatial relationships, and the frontal lobe provides judgment and decision-making. Your conscience (somewhere in your neocortex) prevents you from driving like a maniac. Suddenly, the car in front of you swerves and a two-hundred pound buck appears standing in the middle of the road, antlers and all.

When confronting a frightening "no-eye-contact" situation, animals freeze, remaining completely still for prolonged periods. Inhibiting motion reduces the likelihood of attack (except in this case, the "attacker" is a two-ton SUV barreling down the highway at 60 mph).

At the sight of the deer, nerves from your retina transmit sensory data to the visual thalamus, then the cortex and amygdala deep within the limbic system. Interactions in the cortex occur in milliseconds. Memories about death and the potential damage from hitting a deer register from the amygdala. Lighting-fast motor reflexes such as dropping your phone and clutching the wheel happen simultaneously. Meanwhile a cascade of biochemical events in the limbic system lead to the release of cortisol and chemical messengers that travel to the lower region of the brain and throughout the body. You begin to sweat, feel palpitations, breathe rapidly and if someone took a picture of your face, you'd see that your expression was as frozen as the deer in the headlights.

The activity in your prefrontal lobes just behind your forehead takes place in microseconds. The stress response takes seconds or minutes longer because of the long road it travels throughout the body.

The feeling of a near-accident stays alive in you for years. Memories are the brain's storehouses of information, both learned and significant emotional events like near accidents. In order to create memories, nerve cells are thought to form new protein molecules and new interconnections. No one region of the brain stores all memories because the storage site depends on the type of memory: how to drive a car are memories held in motor areas, while those about smell are held in the olfactory area of the brain. The hippocampus helps the brain select where important memories will be stored. The creation of long-term memories requires attention, repetition, and associative ideas to promote new neural (synaptic) connections, such as those that are formed when practicing a sport or musical instrument. In fact, greater emotional arousal following a learning event enhances a person's retention of that event.[127]

From an evolutionary perspective, stressful memories are stored in the brain on a subconscious level as a throwback to the ancient days when recording details of dangerous events—an encounter with a tiger or snake, for example—would lead to better ways of handling such threats in the future. Your subconscious mind (your sleeping friend or enemy) has great influence over your body. Touch someone, and many times they will have a flashback to a past event in their life. That's because memory is stored in the nerve cells of your body, not just your brain.

As we have seen, your brain and immune system are linked at a biochemical level, continuously signaling each other through the central nervous and immune systems. Your brain interprets the cellular production of emotions, sending this information to the "thinking" part of the brain. Cognition is our ability to process and store information about the world. We are not necessarily conscious of those activities as they occur. As we saw in the example of the near accident with the deer, many aspects of emotion rely on cognition and cognition similarly depends on emotion.[128]

In summary the brain can influence the body; and the body can influence the brain. Scientists discovered that opiate receptors are all over the body, dense in the brain, CNS, spinal cord, ANS, lungs and abdomen. Heavy concentrations of neuropeptides live in the GI tract, skin and muscles, including the heart. More amazingly, your own white blood cells—monocytes—manufacture neuropeptides. The monocytes speak to opiate receptors in the brain; the brain's neuropeptides speak to the body—the blood stream, heart, lungs, GI tract, urinary system, sex organs, muscles, etc. The brain is an associative network throughout the body. When you think negative thoughts, you experience negative emotions and physiological responses like the stress response. Think fear, feel fear. Emotions are biological products of the nervous system.

CHAPTER 7

The Power of Placebo-Nocebo

The great lesson of medical history is that the placebo has always been the norm of medical practice.

– William Osler, M.D.

Placebo is Latin for "I will help." Nocebo is Latin for "I will harm." American medicine has reduced placebo to benchmarks in tests of new drugs and techniques. Contrary to popular belief, a placebo is *not* just a sugar pill. Faith, hope and even the doctor-patient relationship can have powerful placebo or nocebo effects on the mind and healing. Placebo effects are words, rituals or therapies, including surgery and inert medications, to relieve symptoms. Doctors prescribed pharmacological inert substances throughout the first half of the twentieth century to patients to cajole wellness. Explanations for the placebo effect have been debated by the prevailing Western medical orthodoxy for decades. Medicine sees illness predominantly as a disruption of biochemistry; medicine has active ingredients that modify body biochemistry to restore health. By this model, sugar pills should not have a physiological effect. But the evidence is unequivocal: they do.[129]

The placebo effect is huge—anywhere between 35 and 75 percent of patients benefit from taking a dummy pill in studies of new drugs.[131] Red, yellow or orange pills provoke a strong stimulatory or antidepressant effect; blue, purple or green tablets are good for sedation; and white pills are associated with pain relief, especially if they are seen to come from pharmaceutical packaging. Larger tablets have stronger effects than smaller ones, and the more someone takes, the larger the effect. The expectation that medicine will relieve a symptom or complaint leads to improvement in those symptoms. This result has been demonstrated to be so powerful that the FDA now insists that drug companies demonstrate that their products are more effective than placebo before they will receive their approval. Typically, between 35 and 45 percent of people given placebos improve. If a candidate drug outperforms a placebo in two independent studies without serious side effects, the FDA will approve it for use.

The power of a doctor's pronouncement is also profound. The patient-doctor interaction is full of expectations, including the expectation that any treatment prescribed will work. Interpreting a patient's wishes is as much art as science. A bad experience with a doctor can be harmful and even cause nocebo effects. For centuries, doctors followed Hippocrates' injunction to hold out hope to patients, even when it meant withholding the truth. Doctors should not deceive patients, but doctors should relieve pain and suffering through the placebo effect of hope. Today patients may be told more than they need or want to know. When a doctor takes an honesty-is-the-best-policy approach, citing statistics and a poor prognosis, patients may experience despair which causes biochemical depression, furthering their decline. Adverse events and nocebo effects are linked to the information provided to patients. The "word" can cause dramatic consequences.

Scared to Death

A well-liked cardiologist at a prominent university hospital walked past an examining room and said, "T-I!" to the resident physician inside before walking on. "T-I" is a clinical acronym for "tricuspid insufficiency," a disorder involving backward flow of blood across the tricuspid valve, which separates the right ventricle (lower heart chamber) from the right atrium (upper heart chamber), and is a common finding in the general population. But the patient sitting in the examining room understood "T-I" to mean "terminal illness." This was a nocebo—the opposite of the Hippocratic vow to do no harm—and caused temporary heart failure in the patient. A word misinterpreted by the patient almost killed her.

Placebo effects are not restricted to the brain. Changes in brain activity can also influence other physiological functions – corresponding placebo effects have been noted on breathing and heart rate. Cardiopulmonary systems can be inhibited during placebo.[131]

Ten years ago, researchers discovered that women who believed they were prone to heart disease were nearly four times as likely to die as women with similar risk factors who didn't hold such fatalistic views. The higher risk of death, in other words, had nothing to with the usual risk factors—hypertension, cholesterol or diabetes. Instead, it tracked closely with belief. Patients experiencing the nocebo effect presume the worst, health-wise. Already vulnerable when they learn they have a life-threatening disease or chronic illness, patients can feel trapped between reality and possibility and nocebo effects can be a self-fulfilling prophecy.[132]

In medicine, time is a precious commodity. Many doctors, experiencing higher insurance rates and lower returns, can't or won't devote enough time to get to know or educate their patients about therapies outside their medical school purview (a cynic might add their referral relationships with other doctors). Today, the average visit with a doctor lasts a mere six minutes, while the average wait time to see a doctor is forty-five minutes. Even more alarming, one study reports that doctors on average interrupt patients only 18 seconds after they start to talk. A physician has a *70 percent chance*—not 30 percent as taught in medical schools only a few years ago—to help the patient recover or to hurt the patient with a dismissive attitude or misdiagnosis. Health care providers have the opportunity of helping or harming a patient with prescriptions, words, action or inaction.

Health professionals agree that the effectiveness of medical therapy depends on the quality of the relationship between the patient and physician. One of the fathers of medicine, Sir William Osler emphasized patient-physician relationships and the importance of good bedside manner in his revolutionary book, *The Principles and Practice of Medicine*. If a patient doesn't trust his or her doctor enough to share deeply personal problems, the physician will have difficulty helping the person change any unhealthy behaviors.

Remembered Wellness

The experience of pain arises from physiological and psychological factors. All of our thoughts, actions, emotions and memories represent biochemical mechanisms within the brain and body. Messages sent via nerve impulses, hormones in the bloodstream or signaling molecules such as neuropeptides keep cells in constant communication with each other. Belief in a placebo can result in activating biochemical mechanisms to "remember" what it's like to live without pain, and the pain may dissipate. Recent studies using fMRI found that placebos prompt the brain's prefrontal cortex to employ self-distracting strategies.[133] Beliefs can influence mind and body connections that result in physical healing. Even the immune system can be conditioned with conscious effort. After repeated associations between an immunosuppressant and a flavored drink, the drink alone can suppress immune system function. According to Herbert Benson, the biased words "placebo effect" should be changed to "remembered wellness." Remembered wellness is what explains the powerful effect of placebo, and the words "remembered wellness" have a positive connotation.[134]

Placebos decrease the experience of pain. Another study using fMRI revealed that placebos decreased activity in pain-sensitive brain regions, including the thalamus and anterior cingulate cortex, a sort of brain within the brain.[135] The mere expectation of relief from a placebo may be enough to make you feel better. Other studies have shown that the expectation of pain relief activates the brain's most powerful painkilling mechanisms, "mu-opioid" receptors, a part of the class of opiate receptors involved in endogenous pain relief.[136] Mu-opioid receptors have second messengers that seek to reward certain behaviors. The densest amount of mu-opioid receptors is found in the frontal cortex, the more advanced part of the brain. The frontal cortex grows with each vertebrae culminating with humans and doesn't fully develop until early adulthood. We are wired for placebos.

The Expectation of Relief

Placebos are as old as medicine itself. Ancient mystics, medieval alchemists and modern scam artists have profited from magic potions and powders for the ailing, including powdered unicorn horn, which was sold as "strong medicine" for the plague. A hundred years ago, doctors triggered an allergy sufferer to wheeze by showing an artificial rose, proving that visual cues are at least some aspect of the placebo response. Another study involved college students who were told an electric current would be passed through their heads. The researchers warned that the "current" could cause a headache. More than two-thirds of the students reported headaches, although no electricity was used. In one study involving Parkinson's patients, researchers found that placebos released a brain chemical called dopamine, just as a brain exposed to an active drug would do.[137]

The psychological effects of most placebos are short-term. Sir William Osler noted over a century ago, "One should treat as many patients as possible with a new drug while it still has the power to heal."[138]

Perhaps this explains why so many new drugs and surgical devices (not to mention other consumer goods like cars) are more profitable, despite their few enhancements from older, less-expensive products. "In the patient's mind, a prescription is a certificate of assured recovery," said Norman Cousins.[139] It's the doctor's promise of good health—the psychological umbilical cord. The challenge for physicians is balancing: don't overtreat, don't addict—first do no harm.

Doctors are discovering that the definition of placebo differs in many ways, depending on the patient's medical condition, age and beliefs. Mimi Guarneri, M.D., a renowned integrative cardiologist at Scripps Integrative Health Center, wrote about her own creative placebo to help a depressed elderly woman suffering from coronary artery disease. Guarneri had tried the conventional therapies—diet, anti-depressants, exercise and group therapy—but nothing seemed to lift her patient's depression. During one of her visits, she finally sat down and scribbled three words as a prescription for the patient: *A small dog.* The elderly woman followed her doctor's advice and the story ended happily, small dog and all, according to Guarneri.[140]

Psychologist Irving Kirsch believes that the effectiveness of Prozac and similar drugs may be attributed almost entirely to the placebo effect. He analyzed 47 clinical trials of antidepressants and concluded that the expectation of improvement, not adjustments in brain chemistry, accounted for 80 percent of the drugs' effectiveness.[141] In fact, more than half of the trials used by the FDA to approve the six leading antidepressants on the market, the drugs failed to outperform sugar pills, and in the trials that were successful, the advantage of drugs over placebo was slight. Researchers concluded that millions of people may be spending billions of dollars on medicines that owe their popularity to clever marketing.

Placebo effects are more than psychological. Doctors in one study successfully eliminated warts by painting them with a brightly colored, inert dye and promising patients the warts would be gone when the color wore off. In a study of asthmatics, researchers found that they could produce dilation of the airways by simply telling people they were inhaling a bronchodilator, even when they weren't. Patients suffering pain after wisdom-tooth extraction got just as much relief from a fake application of ultrasound as from a real one, so long as both patient and therapist thought the machine was on. Fifty-two percent of the colitis patients treated with placebo in 11 different trials reported feeling better, and 50 percent of the inflamed intestines actually looked better when assessed with a sigmoid scope.[142]

Over 40 years ago, a young Seattle cardiologist named Leonard Cobb conducted a unique trial of a procedure used to treat angina. Surgeons made small incisions in the chest and tied knots in two arteries to increase blood flow to the heart. It was a popular technique (90 percent of patients reported that it helped), but when Cobb compared it with placebo surgeries, the sham operations proved just as successful. The procedure, known as internal mammary ligation, included the chest incision but didn't include tying-off the arteries. The trial was soon abandoned due to ethical concerns.[143]

Faith as Placebo

From the dawn of history, medicine and folklore have been replete with faith placebos. In fact, belief systems the world over have attributed sickness to diabolical or divine interventions, according to medical historian Roy Porter in his book, *The Greatest Benefit to Mankind*.[144] The ancient peoples of Mesopotamia, Egypt and certain Amazon cultures believed that illness was the result of evil spirits possessing the body. Egyptians believed that feelings and thoughts originate in the heart, and the ancient physicians recognized multiple diseases of the "heart-mind." Depression was considered "fever in the heart." Healing methods usually involved worship and spirituality. Medicine, religion and magic were all intertwined with faith.

Shamans in the agrarian cultures of Asia and Native America combined the roles of healer, sage and priest to protect against evil spirits and prevent or cure disease. Early Greek medicine focused on Asclepius, the god of healing. A cult of Asclepius became popular in 300 BC. Worshippers believed that Asclepius, with the help of his daughters Hygeia and Panacea, healed the faithful if they built temples in his name, made sacrifices, and slept in his temples. The original, ancient Hippocratic Oath begins with the invocation "I swear by Apollo the Physician and by Asclepius and by Hygieia and Panacea and by all the gods . . ." Early Romans thought disease was brought on by divine disfavor, and healing occurred when human actions pleased the gods. Religious cures were rare, but magical treatments were common. The Romans used complex concoctions of herbs and animal organ extracts, including snake venom and opium. One popular concoction, "Galen's Theriac," was used well into the nineteenth and early twentieth centuries to treat both physical and mental ailments such as headaches, anxiety, worry and insomnia.

In medieval times, internal diseases were "prevented" by elaborate rituals and "treated" by making the body uninhabitable through torture and starvation. The patient who got better after a bleeding, beating or starving in reality got better because of the natural course of healing or the placebo effect. Spirituality and the soul were considered matters of the Church. And, at the beginning of this period, virtually all of health care in the West was carried out by clergy in hospitals or monasteries that were built and supported by the Church. The practice of medicine didn't become a secular discipline until the end of the sixteenth century when physicians began to be certified by the state. The split between religion and science widened toward the end of this period in Western history.

Death by Diagnosis

Voodoo, a polytheistic religion practiced chiefly by West Indians, still plays an important role in the spiritual life of that culture. The modern voodoo priest or priestess acts as an intermediary between a deity and patient, offering healing through the use of herbs, medicines or faith in their power to heal. Norman Cousins, a journalist who fell gravely ill with a rare disease and wrote about his experiences, described an opportunity to observe a witch doctor while visiting the famed Albert Schweitzer in Africa:

With some patients, the witch doctor merely put herbs in a brown paper bag and instructed the ill person in their use. With other patients, he gave no herbs but filled the air with incantations. A third category of patients he merely spoke to in a subdued voice and pointed to Dr. Schweitzer ... On our way back to the clinic, Dr. Schweitzer explained what had happened. The people who had assorted complaints that the witch doctor was able to diagnose readily were given special herbs to make into brews. Dr. Schweitzer guessed that most of those patients would improve very rapidly since they had only functional, rather than organic, disturbances. Therefore, the "medications" were not really a major factor. The second group had psychogenic ailments that were being treated with African psychotherapy. The third group had more substantial physical problems, such as massive hernias or extrauterine pregnancies or dislocated shoulders or cancerous conditions. Many of these problems required surgery, and the witch doctor was redirecting the patients to Dr. Schweitzer himself.[145]

Witch doctors and medicine men have the mystic powers to rid the body of evil spirits, but they also can instill in people a curse of death. The "evil eye" in some societies is a jealous or harmful glance that can cause physical changes in the believer. In fact, scientists have confirmed that a witch doctor can cause death by convincing the victim that he or she is going to die. Voodoo death—a hex so powerful that the victim of the curse dies of fright—is one of the most extreme examples of the nocebo effect. While many in the scientific community may regard voodoo with skepticism, the idea that gut reactions have biological consequences can't be simply dismissed. Autopsies on patients who have had the nocebo or voodoo effect were found to have myofibrillar heart degeneration. A massive overdose of stress hormones can trigger a cascade of biochemical events, proving fatal. Nocebos can promote illness, even death. The "word" can heal or kill you. I discovered the power of the nocebo effect a few years ago.

I was playing tennis on a Saturday afternoon with a bright blue sky when my pager went off. After finishing the game, I walked off the court and phoned the neurologist on call at the hospital. My doubles partner, Jim bent over to bandage his ankle. He had rolled his ankle on the clay court while lunging after a ball.

"Dr. Kachmann," the voice on the other end of the line said, "we have twenty-eight year old Leslie Chalmers here with a history of seizures. We took an MRI after her CT looked suspicious. Her scan shows a small but malignant-appearing tumor in the right front parietal lobes."

"I see," I said. "Maybe it's a glioblastoma, maybe it's not. What's her neurological status?"

"She's intact but very agitated and inconsolable after I discussed the scan with her."

"I'll be right over."

"Dr. Kachmann? She's creating a lot of chaos in the ER."

"What do you mean?"

"She's wide awake and wanting to be ambulatory ... and won't stop yelling that she wants to die. She recently lost her three-year-old son, and her mother thinks she wants to re-contact him."

The traffic was light—most people spent the hot and humid Indiana summer at the lake on the weekends. I had to think about what I would say to Leslie. Doctors know that somehow they must appeal to their patient's psyche and be the facilitators and midwives of hope, finding just the right words to say. In this case, I not only needed to anticipate the emotional needs of a patient who faced unthinkable odds from a brain tumor, but those of a mother who had just lost a child.

I soon stood outside Leslie's hospital room tracing the light and dark shadows on her brain scan with my finger. The white mass represented a highly malignant brain tumor, a grade four glioblastoma multiforme (GBM). The dark ring circling it was edema (swelling) agitating the adjacent brain tissue. The brain only makes up about 80 percent of the intracranial contents. The other 20 percent is blood and cerebrospinal fluid, which doesn't leave much room for swelling. Edema can lead to elevated pressures within the skull and sometimes irreversible brain damage, but in this case, the swelling was minimal and required no heroic tactics.

When a brain tumor is detected on a CT or MRI scan, I will perform neurosurgery to obtain a biopsy of the tumor for examination by a neuropathologist who can name and grade the tumor. The exact name and grade of the tumor determines the patient's treatment options, and also provides important information about the prognosis or outlook.

Without surgical intervention, patients with glioblastoma multiforme have a five-year survival rate of 3 percent. GBM makes up about 20 percent of all intracranial tumors. Treatment can involve chemotherapy, radiotherapy, and/or surgery, all of which are palliative measures—they don't provide a cure. Leslie was lucky that the tumor was in a non-critical region of the brain. Most GBM quickly infiltrate the brain, often becoming very large before producing symptoms, but Leslie's tumor was still small. In fact, with the appropriate treatment, she had a 95 percent chance of recovery without loss of speech, motor or other neural deficits. Despite the odds in her favor, I was hesitant to discuss the surgery with Leslie. Stress, depression and anxiety prior to surgery are often associated with poor recovery.

"Hi, I'm Dr. Kachmann," I said as I walked into her hospital room. Leslie was laying quietly on her hospital bed, staring out the window. She didn't look like a typical 30 year-old. Her skin was sallow, her cheeks sunken. Her mother began stroking her forehead as I began to describe Leslie's tumor, recommended surgery and favorable prognosis.

Sadness, anger and denial are understandable reactions to a brain tumor diagnosis. Fear of the unknown is a normal response. But sometimes negative attitudes and emotions have a greater impact on mortality than what medical science would anticipate. Or than what I would anticipate. The famous psychologist Karl Menninger once observed that sometimes the diagnosis has a worse affect than the disease. For some, uncertainty is far too unsettling for the mind, and people will go to great lengths to shun it, even if the outcome is fatal, rather than put up with the unknown.

Perhaps what Leslie gave up in her mind, she also gave up in her body, because the stress of her diagnosis was ultimately fatal. Within hours of being admitted, she was in turmoil with her family and the hospital workers. She wouldn't stop shouting that she wanted to die. Could it be the tumor was compromising some part of her brain, making her irrational?

I ordered an emergency head CT and the results were the same— no new mass, bleeding or increased swelling. Later that night, she went into cardiac arrest before we could even begin her treatment for the brain tumor. From a medical standpoint, I couldn't explain Leslie's rapid decline. No "code blue" was initiated upon her request. She was *gone*. What haunts me to this day is that I believe she willed it herself. The will to die is a powerful nocebo.

That night I talked about Leslie's death in the doctor's lounge. No one was willing to concede the nocebo effect, but several doctors accepted the possibility that the emotional devastation from losing a child contributed to the mother's sudden death. In fact, statistics indicate that, on people undergoing surgery who want to die to re-contact a loved one, close to 100 percent of people die.[146] The bigger and more dramatic the patient perceives the intervention to be, the bigger the placebo or nocebo effect.

Natural Relief

Side-effects from drugs cost the US health system more than $177.4 billion a year.[147] If even a small percentage of those costs were caused by patient expectations of harm, addressing the nocebo effect could save millions of taxpayer dollars. Placebo is the body's own ability to right itself—the greatest healing reservoir is your mind and the biochemicals of emotion. The will to live and hope are the most potent drugs. And as I would learn from a cab driver during a trip to Boston, a sense of humor can sustain wellness.

The driver, an Italian-American in his late forties named Gino, was dragging his right leg when attempting to load my luggage in the trunk. I tried to help him but he refused my help. I could tell he had a serious neurological condition. When I introduced myself as a neurosurgeon, he told me he had MS and that he could have applied for disability income but he chose to work. I could see why. On the 20 minute drive to the hotel, he told me one-liners, one right after the other. I was laughing hysterically in the backseat, oblivious to the traffic, noise and pedestrian congestion. He was healing himself: MS is an autoimmune disease, and he had suffered no flare-ups for over 17 years. He was tapping into his body and mind's own immunity through laughter, the best medicine of all. Laughter activates immune T-cells and natural killer cells and increases immunity-boosting interferon. It also reduces the stress hormone, cortisol.[148]

Telling a joke also increases the sense of belonging and distracts the mind from pain. In a recent study of depressed and suicidal senior citizens, patients who demonstrated a sense of humor and interest in others overcame their depression. People with a strong sense of humor tend to remember positive experiences involving people and find a way to let go of negative ones.

Norman Cousins, who watched comedy after comedy while recovering from his near-fatal illness, also wrote about his experience meeting the Spanish musician, Pablo Casals, a virtuoso cello player and conductor. Cousins observed that a highly developed purpose and the will to live were among prime motivators to live a long life. Casals suffered from severe rheumatoid arthritis and emphysema—his back was stooped, hands were swollen and fingers were clenched. Despite his disabilities and pain, Cousins observed a miracle when Casals began to play the piano: his fingers would start to unlock. Eventually he sat up straight and would pound away Bach at the keyboard. Afterwards, Cousins and Casals went for a vigorous walk. Cousins observed that the musician's posture and breathing were normal. But by mid-afternoon, Casals' legs stiffened, his bent posture returned.

Casals was able to cast off his afflictions through the temporary placebo effect of his own drive and creativity.[149] A person's attitude, sense of purpose and beliefs are important to their physical endurance or recovery from injury or illness. Beliefs have a profound effect on mind and body.

Creative Medicine

Johan Strauss conducted orchestras in Vienna throughout the worst period of the late nineteenth-century Prussian Wars—what a placebo in a great time of sorrow. With the proliferation of drugs and procedures that successfully extend life, many doctors have forgotten about the placebo effect. I was reminded of this fact when a good friend and family doctor died recently. His partners who took over his caseload said to me, "He has a lot of very sick patients, but they all seem to be feeling well." Remember, a placebo can be a pill, priest or procedure, but one of the greatest positive forces (outside of your own internal pharmacy) is a compassionate doctor. "The secret of the care of the patient," wrote Dr. Francis W. Peabody in a popular essay for doctors, "is in caring for the patient." Whether you trust your doctor or not makes a huge difference in compliance with treatment. And a good doctor can distract patients from their pain, elicit hope, or build confidence in the human reservoir to overcome adversity in times of suffering. Two of my contemporary heroes in "creative medicine" are Carl A. Hammerschlag, who works with Native Americans in restoring mind, body and spirit and Hunter "Patch" Adams.

Patch is a social activist, professional clown and international diplomat in addition to being a medical doctor. Each year he organizes a group of volunteers from around the world to travel as clowns to bring hope and joy to orphans and the victims of war. Hammerschlag described a scene in war-torn Africa that Patch recently shared with him:

> [Patch] showed us some videotape footage of a little girl with third-degree burns that covered half her body. Her crusted, burned flesh was being treated without anesthetic. I wanted to run away at the sight of such suffering, but the clowns under Patch's tutelage don't run away from anyone. While bandaging the wound, a clown playing a violin stood close by, and let the burned child touch her nose.

If you get too fixated on pills as placebos, you'll miss the larger meaning of placebos. A clown, violin, sense of purpose or even a joke is a placebo. In today's society, loneliness is the source of most people's despair, and if you can reach out and make a difference, they will feel better. You don't have to be a doctor to promote healing in your community. Meanwhile doctors firmly in the fold of evidence-based medicine may want to reconsider offering magic, hope and comfort through the creative art of placebos. The larger meaning of placebos has to do with faith and hope and a physician's compassion and capacity for incorporating those sentiments in the service of the sick.

PART III

The Mind and Specific Illnesses

CHAPTER 8

The Pain Enigma

Pain is temporary. It may last a minute, or an hour, or a day, or a year, but eventually it will subside and something else will take its place. If I quit, however, it lasts forever.

–Lance Armstrong

The enigma of pain, which Albert Schweitzer called "the most terrible of all the lords of mankind," dominates the health care industry. About 50 percent of patients worldwide seek health care for pain-related illness such as backaches, headaches, stomachaches and muscle tension.[150] According to the *Merck Manual*, "pain is an unpleasant sensation signaling actual or possible injury." If Schweitzer were alive today, he might say that some *pain clinics* are the second most terrible lords of mankind.

Millions of Americans are habituated, and a significant number are addicted, because of short-sited methods of treating pain. Within three years of introducing OxyContin, the narcotic became the number one most prescribed pain-killer in the US. Within five years, primary care practitioners were prescribing OxyContin more than oncologists—the specialists who treat cancer.[151] OxyContin has twice the potency of morphine. Government agencies have prosecuted scores of pain doctors who over-prescribe OxyContin to addicts and abusers. In turn, many pain doctors and patients have protested the Drug Enforcement Agency's punitive approach, claiming that it unfairly penalizes pain patients.[152] People who think medicine under treats pain may want to survey psychiatrists who treat the silent epidemic of addiction.

Addiction to prescription and non-prescription drugs is one of the nation's biggest public health problems, costing $524 billion annually, including lost wages and costs to the public health care and criminal justice systems.[153] Patients may think that if a physician prescribes a drug, they're not at risk for becoming an addict. Nothing could be further from the truth. Radio talk-show host Rush Limbaugh's dependence on the painkiller hydrocodone began after an unsuccessful back surgery. Elvis Presley died from massive amounts of pharmaceuticals, prescribed primarily by one physician. Residents in Los Angeles can boast that they have a pain center on almost every corner. American medicine has made an industry out of pain.

What Pain Is

The term "pain" is a subjective experience that typically accompanies a stimulus but also can be psychogenic, occurring without a pain-producing event. Pain is a *perception* spanning multiple pathways within the brain, including sensation, emotion and cognition. Stress-related headaches, lower-back, neck, chest and abdominal pain are common, so common in fact that an estimated 60 to even 90 percent visits to primary doctors are due to such pain. Emotional and physical pain share similar immune system and neural pathways and biochemical processes. In the past, neuroscientists focused on the mechanical basis of pain, and for the most part ignored the emotional, cognitive or psychological aspects.

Psychological stressors (conscious and unconscious) are often difficult to disentangle from pain disorders. In some physical disorders, emotional factors contribute directly or indirectly to the cause; in others, emotional states such as depression or anxiety are the direct result of pathophysiological mind-body conditions such as psychogenic pain. As John Sarno, M.D. notes in *The Divided Mind*, "The emotions we repress are often much more powerful and painful than the emotions we consciously experience."[154]

Acute pain is the most common reason why patients seek medical attention. Acute pain signals are useful and adaptive, warning of danger and the need to escape or seek help. Pain following a broken bone, trauma or surgery triggers a signal to the conscious brain about the presence of harmful stimuli or tissue damage. No test can measure the intensity of pain, although technologies such as x-rays, echocardiograms or nerve conduction studies can help physicians locate the cause of pain. Hospitals and nursing homes include pain as the fifth vital sign to be assessed at the same as blood pressure, pulse, temperature and respiratory rate. The main goal of a health care provider is to diagnose and treat acute pain by clipping the aneurysm, casting the fracture or treating the wound.

Until the mid-seventeenth century physicians believed that pain was felt in the heart. The word pain is thought to derive from the Latin word "poena," meaning punishment. An emotional reaction to a punishment might have been what Aristotle experienced, as he defined pain as an emotional event in the heart. William Harvey, who mapped the circulatory system said, "Just as the king is the first and highest authority in the state," Harvey declared, "so the heart governs the whole body!" René Descartes changed the view of pain, developing the concept of sensory pain pathways. Pain signals traveled from the trauma site to the brain like a rope pulling a bell.

As early as 50 years ago, doctors generally believed that pain traveled directly from the central and peripheral nervous systems to the pain center in your brain—the more severe the pain, the worse the injury. "Nociception" is a neurological term for specific activity in nerve pathways. The work of Scottish anatomist and neurosurgeon Charles Bell laid the groundwork for the concept of nociception, using a telephone exchange model to describe the transmission mechanism for physiological pain.[155] Today researchers studying pain understand that our perception of pain is not directly proportional to the extent of the injury or the intensity of the painful stimuli. Pain research has undergone major changes, from a system level to cellular, sub-cellular and molecular levels.

Understanding how pain works in the body involved studying the chemical signaling system between and within cells. Since the late 1930s, scientists have known that small molecules such as the hormone adrenaline (also called epinephrine) and the nerve chemical, or neurotransmitter, acetylcholine transmit nerve impulses. These molecules act on the outside of the cell by combining with proteins, called receptors, on the cell surface and involve second messengers on the membrane of cells.

A complex system of electrical and chemical exchanges goes into action from the point of injury and the perception of pain. Ultimately, pain results from a series of exchanges among three major components of your nervous system: peripheral nerves, the spinal cord and the brain. Specialized nerve cells within the spinal cord act as gatekeepers that filter fast or slow pain messages on the way to the brain, depending on the stimulus. The pain you feel from spilling a hot cup of coffee is an example of fast pain. Slow pain includes the kind of aching or throbbing pain you experience after spraining your ankle. Some of the factors that increase or decrease the pain experience include memories, focus, and breathing, or emotional states such as fear or joy.

Pain has many complex definitions and categories but there are two main types that we can group according to the source and pain-detecting neurons: nociceptive and neuropathic. Arthritic pain, including rheumatoid arthritis, osteoarthritis and even fibromyalgia are types of inflammatory pain with varied pathophysiological mechanisms.

Nociceptive pain can be divided into two separate categories: visceral and somatic. The differences are important for understanding the origin of the pain and how to manage or treat it. Most aching, sharp, or throbbing pain is nociceptive pain. A familiar experience of nociceptive pain is the frustrating pain of stubbing your toe at the foot of the bed in the middle of the night. Your toes are loaded with nerve fibers and nociceptors, receptors that detect actual or potential tissue damage. Millions of nociceptors exist throughout your body in your skin, bones, joints and muscles and in the protective membrane around your internal organs, but they are abundant in areas prone to injury, such as your little toes. When the electrical and chemical signals sent by nociceptors reach a processing area in the spinal cord called the dorsal horn, a signal is immediately sent back along motor nerves to the original site of the pain, triggering the muscles to contract, a reflex reaction that helps prevent permanent damage.

Reflexes are responses to stimuli that do not require conscious thought and consequently, they occur more quickly than reactions that require thought processes. Most reflexes go completely unnoticed because they don't involve a visible and sudden movement. Body functions such as heart rate, digestion or blood pressure, for example, are all regulated by autonomic reflexes. A reflex action often involves a very simple nervous pathway within the spinal cord called a reflex arc. With the withdrawal reflex such as jerking your hand back from a hot grill, the reflex action withdraws the affected part before you're even aware of the pain. Many reflexes are mediated in the spinal cord without going to the higher brain centers which avoids the delay of routing signals through the brain. When I perform a neurological exam, I check innate reflexes by tapping the tendon below your kneecap.

Deep within your brain, the thalamus quickly forwards pain messages simultaneously to three specialized regions of the brain: the physical sensation region (somatosensory cortex), the emotional feeling region (limbic system) and the thinking region (frontal cortex). Modern electrophysiology has been used to demonstrate the critical roles of synaptic plasticity in pain processing in the spinal cord and the brain. Only when the brain processes the signal and interprets it as pain do you become *conscious* of the pain. Nociceptive pain also causes a rise in heart rate, blood pressure and breathing rate, as well as changes in behavior—a contorted face or exclamation (which in good taste cannot be repeated here).

Endorphins released from the limbic system help reduce the intensity of pain. If you recall from the section on the science of emotions, endorphins are small-chain peptides that activate our endogenous opioid receptors embedded in cell membranes. Opiate agonists bind to the receptors to initiate their pain-relieving effects. The highest density of opiate receptors is found in the limbic system of the brain which influences the formation of important memories by integrating emotional states with stored memories of physical sensations like pain or ecstasy. Functional imaging has revealed central areas related to pain processing such as areas coding behavioral learning and memory and, more significantly, it has now become possible to see the alteration of these signaling pathways under chronic pain conditions. Emotions and memories meld together in the mind and body, protecting us from harm but sometimes backfiring with unwanted behavioral responses.

Acute pain from trauma is a barometer that warns us about tissue damage. Pain within the cutaneous tissues (skin) or deep tissues (bones or joints) from an accident or surgery is generally within the nociceptive subtype of somatic pain. Surface, localized pain from something like a paper cut is somatic. Visceral pain is the subtype of nociceptive pain that involves internal organs and tends to be episodic and poorly localized (diffuse). "Viscera" refers to the internal areas of the body enclosed within a cavity. For example, if you experience a sudden unbearable headache with neck pain, especially when lifting, coughing or straining, I would suspect an aneurysm. Uncomfortable pressure, fullness or squeezing pain in the center of the chest, sometimes spreading to the shoulders, neck or arms could signal a heart attack. In either case, call 911.

Chronic Pain

Pain is a lucrative business. The worldwide painkiller market was worth $50 billion in 2005 and is expected to increase to $75 billion by 2010 and $105 billion by 2015. The National Institute on Drug Abuse and the National Institute on Alcohol Abuse and Alcoholism are studying, or financing studies on, more than 200 addiction medications to treat an estimated 20 million drug addicts in the United States. Addiction vaccines are already in development. Neuroscientists studying addiction have found that painkillers cause an increase in the amount of dopamine secreted between neurons, leading to feelings of euphoria. With repeated drug use, the brain reprograms itself and responds to pain by reducing the release of dopamine and dopamine receptors and becoming more dependent on artificial means of stimulating the reward system.[156]

By some estimates, chronic pain affects nearly 100 million Americans from such varied causes as diabetes, cancer and fibromyalgia. The financial cost of chronic pain is in the same range as cancer and cardiovascular disease with backaches topping the list at $50 to $100 billion in health care costs and lost wages. A recent study found that prescribing opioids to patients with chronic disabling back pain doubled the risk that the patient would be out of work and the likelihood that a patient would engage in excessive healthcare-seeking behavior.[157]

Long-term or chronic pain typically lasts more than six months, despite treatment and coping efforts, and has no protective role for the body. "Chronic pain is a disease of the central nervous system that may or may not correlate with any tissue damage but involves an errant reprogramming in the brain and spinal cord," according to Sean Mackey, a neuroscientist at Stanford University's Pain Center and one of the leading experts on pain research.[158] As I discussed in the section on neuropathic pain, altered electrical and chemical nerve signals may cause pain to drag on long after the injury has healed.

Clifford Woolf, M.D. of Harvard Medical School, another leading expert on pain, investigates the way in which functional, chemical and structural plasticity of neurons contributes to pain. He identified a genetic variation in some humans associated with lower pain sensitivity, proving that we inherit the extent to which we feel pain, both under normal conditions and after damage to the nervous system. "Individuals who say they feel less pain are not just stoics but genuinely have inherited molecular machinery that reduces their perception of pain. This difference results not from personality or culture, but real differences in the biology of the sensory nervous system."[159] For anyone who suffers with chronic pain, mind-body medicine can make a big difference, offering choices through a multidisciplinary approach that integrates conventional pain-relief treatments with scientifically-based complementary therapies.

Types of Chronic Pain

Neuropathic pain is caused by abnormalities in the nerves, spinal cord, or brain. For example, arachnoiditis is a pain disorder caused by the inflammation of the membranes that surround and protect the nerves of the spinal cord. Arachnoids can become inflamed because of an irritation from chemicals, infection, spinal injury, chronic compression of spinal nerves, or complications from spinal surgery or other invasive spinal procedures.

The perception of neuropathic pain is real, whether or not harm has occurred or is occurring. Robyn is a 42-year-old woman who feels burning arm pain from even a light touch as a result of an injury from a car accident several years ago. Her injury has healed, but the nervous system continues to misinterpret signals that should not be painful. In the past, doctors may have diagnosed her pain as psychosomatic. Current research suggests that cytokines, the in-between cell messengers which play a major role in a variety of immunological, inflammatory and infectious diseases, may be involved in the pathology of arachnoiditis. Blocking cytokines has provided relief in some patients.

Multiple Sclerosis (MS) is the most common cause of central neuropathic pain. Autonomic firing of pain impulses can result in chronic, continuous pain in patients while other MS patients may develop hyperplasia (exaggerated pain). The symptoms are varied and can include visual problems and fatigue. Central neuropathic pain can be worse at night or non-active days. Patients with MS will have periods of remission, sometimes for years, and then may experience flare-ups and need to be ready with a plan to remedy it. While the mechanisms of MS are under study, scientists now know that inflammatory and autoimmune diseases such as MS and arthritis are associated with a communication breakdown between the brain and immune system. The immune system mistakenly attacks and destroys the protective sheath around neurons, disrupting communication throughout the brain and spinal cord. In individuals with mild fatigue from MS, non-pharmacological treatments including yoga, aerobic exercise and cooling therapy helps.

When Nancy Davis was diagnosed with MS at age 33, her neurologist told her to go home and "go to bed ... forever." Now an advocate for MS, founder of the Center Without Walls (a medical research foundation), and author of *Lean on Me*, Davis teaches people how to move beyond the negative aspects of the disease and focus on what they personally can and will do to improve their health. She urges people to "follow your bliss," and ask yourself, "What has prevented me form living out my passion?" Davis has found homeopathy, acupuncture and osteopathy to be useful for her MS pain.

The third type of pain is neuropathic and results from abnormal nerve functions or direct damage to a nerve such as entrapment neuropathy, more widely known as carpal tunnel syndrome (CTS). Pain detecting nerves in the periphery can suffer direct damage, resulting in neuropathic pain and changes in the brain's somatosensory system which processes touch, pain, pressure, temperature, and joint and muscle position. Acupuncture, a somatosensory conditioning stimulus, has shown promise in inducing beneficial cortical plasticity. Other examples of neuropathic pain include phantom limb pain, diabetic neuropathy and shingles—all which can cause severe pain.

Another illustration of the power of the mind in the body is that people can suffer with severe pain, even when the body part is no longer part of the body. Military field surgeons in Iraq know that if they administer nerve blockers immediately after a soldier's limb injury they can reduce the risk of phantom pain—the debilitating neuropathic pain amputees often feel in their stumps years after combat. Nerves severed in an amputation or accident may cluster into a mass called a neuroma that causes severe burning and aching and intermittent shooting pain. Neuropathic pain can affect mastectomy patients as well. More recently, neurologist V.S. Ramachandran has proven that phantom limb sensations could be due to neural misfiring in the somatosensory cortex of the brain. His book, *Phantoms in the Brain*, describes the power of the mind in this bizarre syndrome:

I placed a coffee cup in front of John and asked him to grab it with his phantom limb. Just as he said he was reaching out, I yanked the cup away.

"Ow!" he yelled. "Don't do that!"

"What's the matter?"

"Don't do that," he repeated. "I had just got my fingers around the cup handle when you pulled it. That really hurts!"

Hold on a minute. I wrench a real cup from phantom fingers and the person yells, ouch! The fingers were illusory, but the pain was real—indeed, so intense that I dared not repeat the experiment.[160]

Often a phantom limb is painful because it feels stuck in an uncomfortable or unnatural position, and the patient cannot move it. Ramachandran argues that there is an indisputable link between neurology and psychology in his acclaimed book, *The Emerging Mind*. In order to retrain the brain, and thereby eliminate the "learned" paralysis and pain, Ramachandran and his associates developed a mirror box as therapy:

The patient places his or her good limb into one side, and the stump into the other. The patient then looks into the mirror on the side with good limb and makes "mirror symmetric" movements, as a symphony conductor might, or as we do when we clap our hands. Because the subject is seeing the reflected image of the good hand moving, it appears as if the phantom limb is also moving. Through the use of this artificial visual feedback it becomes possible for the patient to "move" the phantom limb, and to unclench it from potentially painful positions.[161]

One of my associates, a neurologist, treated a young man who almost cut off his right hand while hoisting up his two-ton fishing boat. The cable on his automatic boat lift snapped, whipping and severing his right thumb, index and middle fingers. Years later, whenever he moved his right hand he had the painful sensation that his thumb and fingers were hyper-extended as they were when his fingers were cut off. We can acquire novel insights into the functions of the normal brain by studying neurological diseases and syndromes.

The Epidemic of Diabetic Pain

Today 65 percent of US adults, age 20 years and older, are overweight and 31 percent are obese. Severe obesity prevalence is now 5 percent of the American population.[162] Because diabetes is a consequence of poor eating habits and obesity, I see more diabetic neuropathy than any other type of pain. More than four million Americans live with nerve pain that can feel like walking on broken glass or electric shocks. About 50-75 percent of non-traumatic amputations are due to diabetic neuropathy.[163] Diabetes is also the leading cause of blindness. Exercise and tight control of blood sugar levels prevents the development of complications. Most of those who have diabetes have Type 2, in which obesity and poverty are key contributors, especially among African Americans and Hispanics, who are disproportionately stricken.

According to the American Diabetes Association, 41 million people in the US have pre-diabetes, i.e., insulin resistance and probably don't even know it. While glucose elevations may be below the threshold of diabetes, insulin resistance increases the risk for heart disease, retinopathy and kidney dysfunction. Regular visits to a nutritionist are not typically covered by insurance, but your regular physician can check for insulin resistance and recommend dietary changes before the disease progresses. Unfortunately, insurance reimbursements are easier when the disease is far along, and the patient needs amputation of toes or limbs. The direct and indirect costs of diabetes are nearly $132 billion a year.[164]

A family doctor recently referred a patient to me with severe diabetic neuropathic shoulder and arm pain. Robert was a 54-year-old, non-compliant diabetic with an average blood sugar of 300 plus who smoked, didn't follow a diet, and refused to exercise. His doctor said he was belligerent and demanding. When I met Robert, I could tell he was miserable. He nodded to me when I came into the examining room then continued rubbing his shoulder. Robert was a mountain of a man, tipping the scale around 280 pounds. He lived on a fixed disability income, had no immediate family in the area and used a portable oxygen machine.

During our interview, I discovered that Robert and I have something in common: we both enjoyed playing the piano. I try to play the piano for twenty minutes each morning before work.

(Practicing the piano helps promote brain growth as you grow older). Robert and I discussed music scores we preferred and promised to exchange CDs during our next visit together. As we spoke about something he liked, I could see his pain lighten in front of my eyes, and in that moment, his personality changed. He became more friendly and receptive to my advice.

"Robert," I said, "what are we going to do about your pain?"

We discussed diet, exercise, stress and pain reduction techniques, breathing exercises, and finally, pain medication. One month later, unlike his previous office visit, which was consumed with pain management strategies, we spoke mainly about our mutual music hobby. Building a relationship with Robert was mutually beneficial; it distracted him from his chronic pain, and motivated me to practice the piano. While diabetic neuropathy is incurable and often resistant to conventional treatment, strict diet help prevents progression; and massage, acupuncture, hypnosis and biofeedback provide temporary relief. The pain can also be helped by keeping busy and focusing attention on something else—like playing the piano.

In osteoarthritis (OA), the degree of pain can vary from mild, moderate to debilitating. About 100 different types of OA affect nearly 21 million people in America, accounting for 25 percent of visits to primary care physicians, and half of all anti-inflammatory prescriptions. An estimated 80 percent of the US population will have imaging (radiograph) evidence of OA by age 65, although only 60 percent will actually feel symptoms of pain, swelling and stiffness.[165] The most important advice I give to people suffering from OA is that degenerative disc or joint disease is benign—a normal part of aging. Many common pain disorders that are thought of as structural in origin also have stress or psychological components. OA can be made worse by certain ways of thinking, negative emotions and lifestyle choices such as smoking which contributes to osteoporosis.

Research suggests that some combination of stress management, coping skills training, and cognitive restructuring and relaxation therapy may be appropriate complimentary treatments for chronic pain from OA. A low fat vegetarian diet can reduce arthritis symptoms by increasing antioxidants. Be careful when choosing herbal supplements for osteoarthritis—many are expensive and harmful, and be sure to ask your doctor about side-effects if you're taking several medications.

Collagen hydrolysate, ginger extract, and vitamins C and D3 have been scientifically proven to help with OA. Acupuncture, yoga and Tai Chi seem to provide improvement in function and pain relief.[166]

A herniated disc is a common cause of lower back pain related to OA. Discs are flat, plate-like structures between the vertebrae (back bones) in the spinal column. They have a tough covering over a soft, gelatinous inside and their purpose is to cushion the back bones and allow the back to flex. A hernia is a tear in the covering of the disc that allows the soft interior to bulge out. In most cases, a herniated disc will heal on its own with a couple of days of bed rest, over-the-counter pain relievers to help with the discomfort, and anti-inflammatory medications. If the disc has fragmented, I may recommend surgery to remove the pieces of the disc that are compressing the nerve. A variety of mind-body therapies, e.g., imagery, when employed pre-surgically, can improve recovery time and reduce pain.

Unlike OA, which results from the normal wear and tear of the cartilage that caps the bones in your joints, rheumatoid arthritis (RA) is a systemic disease that can affect various parts of the body including blood vessels, organs and muscles. Like multiple sclerosis, RA is a chronic pain condition associated with an impaired hormonal stress response which promotes inflammation. The exact cause of RA is unknown, but scientists believe the body's immune system attacks the membrane tissue that lines the joints. In general, RA affects women twice as often as men. With RA, the membrane that protects and lubricates joints becomes inflamed, causing pain and swelling. Joint erosion may follow. Infection which causes a defect in the immune system's ability to distinguish self from foreign molecules, or physical and emotional effects, stress and improper diet could play a role in the disease.

Cytokines, the in-between immune cell messengers which we discussed in the pathology of arachnoiditis, may be responsible for the inflammatory pain associated with RA. Treatment includes disease-modifying anti-rheumatic drugs, (which are critical in the early stages of the disease to prevent permanent joint damage), and several non-standard therapies that help with joint mobility and pain relief, including yoga, hypnosis, deep breathing, Tai Chi, and chiropractic and visualization techniques. I also recommend fish oil supplements for many of my patients who have inflammatory disease. The body can use fish oil (omega-3s) to make substances that reduce inflammation.

Even healthy people should eat omega-3 fatty acids from fish and plant sources to protect their hearts and brains. Research suggests that fish oil decreases the risk of arrhythmias and lowers triglyceride levels and the growth rate of atherosclerotic plaque, all of which protects you from sudden death, heart attack and stroke.

About 28 million Americans suffer from severe migraines that leave them temporarily unable to function at work, at home or at play while others suffer milder forms. Migraine headaches are now recognized to stem from neural changes in the brain and the release of inflammatory peptides that in turn constrict blood vessels. The inflammatory peptides sensitize nerve fibers that then respond to innocuous stimuli, like blood vessel pulses, causing the pain of migraine even before these vessels dilate. The WHO ranks migraines among the most disabling illnesses. Employers lose about $13 billion a year in lost productivity, with another $1 billion spent on health care for migraines.

Cancer Pain

For people living with chronic or life-threatening illness due to cancer, mind-body medicine can transform the physical, emotional, and spiritual dimensions of their lives. Cancer pain may be short-lived or long-lasting, mild or severe, or affect one or a few organs, bones or organ systems. Each patient's pain is unique. Pain from the tumor, cancer treatment such as surgery, chemotherapy or radiotherapy, or even another condition may contribute to cancer pain. Therapies such as meditation, yoga, biofeedback or even prayer rituals can help alleviate stress, reduce pain and anxiety, manage symptoms, and promote a feeling of well-being during cancer treatment. I try to pray with my patients undergoing any kind of brain surgery.

Complex Chronic Pain

In my line of work, there is an epidemic of musculoskeletal pain. An injury or trauma, particularly in the upper spinal region, may trigger the kind of chronic back pain in which five million Americans face each day. Chronic pain of this type can impact all areas of a person's life and is often associated with psychological and social problems.

146 • Welcome To Your MindBody

Perhaps two-thirds of people suffering from chronic pain have symptoms that standard diagnostics such as blood tests, biopsies, x-rays, scans or scopes cannot explain. Pain of this sort is a medical enigma, meaning it has no obvious trigger (tear, tumor or nerve damage), and no organic disease explains it. Stress, emotional factors and the way the brain and nervous system process pain are ubiquitously interrelated with complex chronic pain syndromes. The pain may develop for no apparent reason, or an intense psychological event may trigger it.

One recent March evening, I received a call that a 42-year-old woman, Heather, had arrived in the Emergency Room requiring urgent neurological care. Heather was an active woman, who had become an expert in the culinary arts and gardening, but her back pain started to limit her activity and she began, in her words, "to feel her age." She had the kind of unexplained back pain that afflicts at least 70 percent of Americans.[167]

Six years ago, after complaining of unrelenting back pain, Heather's primary care doctor performed a magnetic resonance imaging (MRI) scan and diagnosed her with degenerative disc disease, a common finding that reflects the normal process of aging. Her doctor advised her to rest and treated her with a series of trigger point injections (a local anesthetic with steroid). By the end of two years, Heather had received 82 injections and had given up exercise and gardening, but continued to, in her words, "cook and put on the pounds."

The next year, her doctor referred her to a local pain clinic where over a few months she was injected 60 more times and finally prescribed Vicodin, a potent pain medication. She said she had tried to exercise but discovered that her back pain was compounded by headaches from the habituation of pain medications. Now, and according to her doctor's referral notes, she became irritable and depressed about her unrelenting pain, demanding an anti-depressant, sleep aid, pain patch and more and more tests to search for the cause of her increasing pain and debilitation.

Over a six year period, Heather had 13 imaging tests and 142 trigger injections, was addicted to narcotics, lost her thick mane of long hair, and had lost over 60 pounds. When I met her, she was curled-up on a hospital gurney and clearly in pain and asked me to examine her without the overhead lights.

"Dr. Kachmann," she said, "I was a yoga instructor until my twelve-year-old daughter died."

I felt sick to my stomach. As I thought about what she said and read her history, a slow, seething anger rose up from my gut, a fire that helped fuel the creation of mind-body lectures which led to this book and the Kachmann Mind Body Institute. Heather was living proof that short-sited medical care contributes directly or indirectly to the patient's loss of control, reduced activity, addiction, depression and eventual disability. When we experience any pain, it exists in both the mind and body. We cannot separate the physical and psychological affects any situation has on us.

A popular theory espoused by John Sarno, M.D. is that psychogenic pain acts as a diversion from threatening emotions such as grief, resentment, anger or anxiety, causing muscle ischemia (lack of blood flow), tension and chronic pain. Although it can be both debilitating and extremely painful, it involves no tissue or nerve damage and can disappear quickly without any permanent residual effects. According to Sarno, most back pain of this type has its roots in emotional stress from certain personality traits, and thus the mind, rather than the body, should be treated to address the symptoms. When it comes to psychogenic pain, no longer is the pain viewed as just the symptom of another disease, but as an illness unto itself. Studies have shown that factors such as anxiety, post-traumatic stress, depression and even loneliness play a key role in many psychogenic pain syndromes. The *Merck Manual* defines psychogenic pain as:

> ... a disorder in which pain in one or more anatomic sites is exclusively or predominantly caused by psychological factors ... Any part of the body may be affected, but the back, head, abdomen, and chest are probably the most common. The pain may be acute or chronic. There may be an underlying physical disorder that explains the pain but not its severity, its duration, nor the degree of resulting disability.[168]

Psychogenic pain syndromes may be due to alterations in the regulation of neurotransmitters such as serotonin, which influences depression, migraines and gastrointestinal distress; or substance P, a brain chemical associated with pain, stress and anxiety. Although the electrophysiological and biochemical mechanisms behind psychogenic pain are varied and complex, the idea is straightforward: your activity, emotions and thoughts influence your brain, immune and nervous system, and in turn, your brain affects your perception of pain. We all consciously and unconsciously control our brain for every activity we initiate, every thought we have, and every emotion or sensation we experience. Some of the factors that modulate pain include attention or distraction, anxiety, fear or depression which disrupts blood flow to the brain, and may also contribute to the discomfort and fatigue of complex chronic pain syndromes.

Enigmatic pain is often misunderstood or considered "all in your head." The pain is real. The mechanisms underlying the pain, however, differ. Pain is a complex, adaptive network involving several brain modules that transmit information back and forth. Psychogenic pain syndromes may involve either an overactive immune system, pain-perception circuit or an underactive pain-modulation circuit.

Several studies have shown that women tend to have a more active pain-perception circuit in the brain. In a recent pain study, male and female volunteers were asked to dunk their arm in warm water for two minutes before plunging the same arm into a vat of icy water for two minutes or until they could stand the pain no longer. Women felt pain much sooner than the men and were able to endure it for far less time, supporting previous research on differing pain thresholds between women and men.[169]

As Louann Brizendine, M.D. points out in *The Female Brain*, women have finely tuned emotional sensitivity—gut feelings that men often lack. The neurobiology of women's intuition, the intense physical sensation that something's wrong, uses the same neural pathways as pain perception. Brain anatomy and possibly estrogen pump up women's ability to feel both physical and emotional pain (and pleasure). Differences in metabolism and fluctuations in hormones that influence the activity of nerves (neuroendocrine) may also play a role. According to imaging studies, the areas of the brain that track gut feelings, the anterior cingulate cortex is larger in females. The anterior cingulate is critical for forethought, judging and integrating emotions and memories. In general, women are gifted at quickly assessing the intentions of others based on behavioral cues. The downside is that they may "pay" for their mind-reading abilities with a lower pain threshold.

Abnormalities of the autonomic (sympathetic) nervous system could be a factor, too. If you recall from the section on the stress response, our autonomic nervous system has both the sympathetic and parasympathetic systems. Your sympathetic nervous system releases norepinephrine and influences the release of epinephrine from the adrenal gland during the stress response. The sympathetic nervous system also controls unconscious functions such as heart rate, blood vessel contraction, sweating and intestinal movements. When stress hormones remain in your body for long durations on a daily basis for years, damage can occur to your nervous and immune systems.

Complex chronic illnesses involve a web of causality with many factors that are not linked to each other in a linear, predictable manner. Chronic fatigue syndrome (CFS) and fibromyalgia are leading examples of complex chronic illnesses. Both conditions involve the immune, circulatory, digestive and nervous systems, which interact with each other in complex ways. The immune systems of persons afflicted with CFS churn out abnormally high levels of the hormones normally responsible for stimulating immune cells into action. These hormones can create a deep sense of fatigue. Individuals with CFS can also have serious problems with memory and concentration, pain and digestion.

Fibromyalgia is a chronic disorder characterized by widespread muscular aching, stiffness and pain at specific sites called "tender points" located in the neck, back and extremities. It is the most common cause of general muscular pain affecting women in their early twenties. While the pain may feel localized to muscles, ligaments or tendons, the body doesn't show any signs of disease. The pain occurs when the brain encounters disturbance while processing normal nerve impulses. Fibromyalgia sufferers can also experience CFS-like symptoms.

A labyrinth of factors may contribute to the two complex illnesses. While each factor by itself may not be sufficient to cause the illness, a multiplicity of factors establish an insidious pattern of chronic symptoms. With a sudden trauma or injury, extreme or chronic stress, environmental toxins, possibly certain germs and a person's genetic vulnerabilities, the factors all join together to wreak havoc, and a complex chronic illness results. Psychological stress, such as repressed fear or anger, may contribute to the illness. Under stress, the immune system "talks" to the brain to trigger survival-oriented sickness responses, including fever, sleep, generalized suppression of behavior and pain, all of which may contribute to the symptoms of CFS and fibromyalgia.

Activated immune cells associated with peripheral nerves and activated nerve cells within the spinal cord contribute to the creation and maintenance of pain enhancement. Activated immune cells alter the function of peripheral nerves via the release of a variety of pro-inflammatory substances. Similarly, immune activation within the spinal cord enhances pain by increasing the release of "pain" transmitters from sensory afferents and increasing excitability of pain transmission neurons. Neuropeptides, such as opioids are also involved in immune system processes related to inflammation and pain. Insidiously, nerve cells become progressively more activated in response to chronic opioids, and contribute to decreasing pain-relieving efficacy by the release of pro-inflammatory cytokines.

These recent research findings are leading to the development of novel strategies for controlling pathological pain conditions, including MS, arthritis and complex pain syndromes. One such strategy includes guided imagery intervention. In a study published January 2006 in the *Journal of Alternative and Complementary Medicine*, one group of patients received standard medical care, plus guided-imagery audiotapes. The other group received only standard care. Compared with the controls, the patients who participated in guided imagery were better able to perform activities of daily living and had a greater sense of being able to manage their pain and other symptoms. The pain didn't change, but the ability to cope with it did.

Fibromyalgia isn't progressive, crippling or life-threatening. Treatments and self-care steps like stretching, yoga and meditation can improve symptoms and restore health. Chiropractic care has been successfully used to treat fibromyalgia. Massage therapy is one of the oldest methods of health care still in practice to help fibromyalgia. Massage uses different manipulative techniques to move your body's muscles and soft tissues. The therapy aims to improve circulation in the muscle, increasing the flow of nutrients and eliminating waste products. Another complementary therapy I recommend is acupuncture. Acupuncture is a Chinese medical system based on restoring normal balance of life forces by inserting very fine needles through the skin to various depths. According to Western theories of acupuncture, the needles cause changes in blood flow and levels of neurotransmitters in the brain and spinal cord. In a recent study, acupuncture significantly improved symptoms of fibromyalgia.

Tension Myositis

Tension Myositis (TMS) is a condition in which chronic, excessive emotional stress causes physical pain. Most often this pain occurs in the back, neck, shoulders and buttocks, but it may appear in other parts of the body as well. According to John Sarno, MD, the physiological reason for the pain is decreased blood flow, causing oxygen deprivation in the affected area of the body, typically muscles, nerves, tendons or ligaments.

Chronic attacks of pain, fear of recurrence and failure to find treatment characterizes TMS. People with this chronic pain syndrome may say, "Every time I lift I feel pain." While the neurobiology of pain doesn't work that way, many people are reluctant to accept that TMS is a functional illness within their body's own healing power to overcome.

TMS is a mind-body syndrome, in that it is a physical condition whose ultimate cause is psychological. However, having TMS does not make you a hypochondriac or malingerer. TMS is real pain, with an immediate cause that is both real and physical. It is certainly not an indication of "mental illness." In fact, TMS patients are often highly responsible and successful individuals.

TMS is a "distraction pain syndrome" of sorts, a very painful strategy for staying sane in a crazy-making world. As we have discussed, many things cause tension, including "external" stressors such as financial, familial or health concerns and "internal" stressors such as conscientiousness, perfectionism, or a need to excel. Your conscious emotions are only the tip of the iceberg; the subconscious mind dominates the mental apparatus, including thoughts, emotions and will. Physical defenses are good and grab attention, camouflaging the negative subconscious emotions.

Sarno claims that simply educating the mind about TMS is the most important step in the process to make it go away. However, he advises patients that they should first have a thorough physical examination by a qualified physician. This is done primarily to exclude more serious conditions, such as fractures, tumors, or infections that require conventional care and it also can identify symptoms that are typical of TMS, such as certain tender points that become painful when pressed.

The remaining steps to recovery, according to Sarno include to first, "Repudiate the physical and acknowledge the psychological aspect," which includes moving around and resuming normal activity as much as you can bear without worrying about "re-injury" (easier said than done). Keep this in mind: with TMS the only thing wrong with your back is that it hurts.

The second step is to "drive the concept to your unconscious" by repeatedly focusing on exactly what your unconscious mind is attempting to repress—the sources of your anger. Sarno and his colleague David Schechter, M.D. developed a 30-day, daily journal called "The Mind-Body Workbook" to record emotionally significant events and make correlations between them their physical pain. The point is to become aware of repressed emotions, which usually involves identifying their sources. The three major sources include: 1) one's childhood; 2) personality type (self-critical, overly responsible, often perfectionist, prone to guilt); and 3) life's challenges. Once the mind understands the trick it is playing on itself, it gives up the ruse, and the symptoms will usually disappear after daily repetition.

The most common misdiagnoses of TMS—degenerative discs and bulging discs—are equally prevalent in the general population as they are among those in chronic pain. In fact, most back pain, (an estimated 85 percent of cases) has no known physiological cause, beyond the persistent muscle tension that is usually associated with it. In many cases, back pain tends to move around, up and down the spine, or from side to side, which is not typical of pain caused by a physical deformity or injury. According to medical research cited by Sarno, psychosocial factors, such as on-the-job stress and dysfunctional family relationships, correlate much more closely with back pain than structural abnormalities revealed in x-rays and other medical imaging scans. This may be why back pain is more prevalent in industrialized countries, where more people have sedentary jobs, than in developing countries, where more people live by "backbreaking" hard labor. TMS also peaks at midlife, during the "age of responsibility," and diminishes to the point of being relatively rare among the elderly. If it were due to degenerative structural conditions in the spine, one would think that it would simply get worse with age. Treatment strategies such as "The Mind-Body Workbook," in addition to complementary therapies such as massage, yoga and tai chi or chi gong, will help resolve the pain of TMS with less expense than conventional medical techniques.

Coping with Chronic Pain

Whatever the cause, chronic pain can be so intractable that it becomes a continuous presence, a constant psychic companion which often sets the stage for the emergence of a complex set of physical and psychosocial changes that increases the burden of the patient, including:

- immobility and muscle wasting;
- depression of the immune system and increased disease susceptibility;
- insomnia;
- poor nutrition and appetite;
- addiction to pain medication;
- dependence on caregivers;
- overuse of health care systems;
- unemployment and disability insurance;
- social isolation;
- loss of sexual interest;
- anxiety and depression[170]

Current medical concepts of pain are mechanistic, localized and empirical, and tend to neglect or separate the psychological components. But pain is a subjective and personal experience influenced by intimate and broader social and physical environments. All pain is physiological *and* psychological. Today, pain researchers are not only focusing on identifying the genetic and biology mechanisms that underlie pain, but they're also investigating the psychological factors, with the goal of developing new and better treatment strategies.

Before performing a spinal tap—a diagnostic procedure to collect a sample of cerebrospinal fluid (CSF) for analysis—I never use the words "needle" or "spine," and advise the medical assistants in the room to do the same. Why? Because patient anxiety during a lumbar puncture can lead to increased CSF fluid pressure, especially if the patient holds their breath or tenses their muscles. Shifting attention away from anxiety and projecting the stimulus as a *neutral* sensory experience rather than one that is damaging or frightening, can help lessen the experience of pain.

Pain Placebos and Nocebos

Our emotional state skews our perception of pain by seeking out memories that match our mind-set. Doctor's can influence patient's perception of pain over the long term—remember placebo, nocebo. Richard Walker, M.D., a British expert in pain management, illustrates how a doctor can dramatically influence a patient's perception of back pain in the following story contrasting two patients with the same problem but different outcomes.

Patient A consults Doctor A, who says the pain is due to an acute soft tissue sprain, the body has tremendous powers of healing, it's a self limiting problem, no real harm has been done, keep as active as you can within the pain, and then you will have a 90 percent chance of it all settling down on its own without treatment in two weeks.

Patient B, who has a similar condition as Patient A, consults Doctor B, who says, you've damaged your back while lifting at work, the X-ray you had yesterday shows early osteoarthritis, rest if it hurts too much, your pain is a warning that you've overdone things, it can only can worse with age, there is no cure for spinal arthritis.

You can see that these two patients will come out of the doctor's visit with completely differing ideas about their back pain. Their doctors have instilled different beliefs into their minds. From now on their behaviors in relation to their back pain are going to be completely different:

Patient A will have positive beliefs around his back pain, expecting that the pain will go away on its own, and that maintaining normal activities will be good for his back. It is quite likely that this patient will recover fully and go on to have a normal lifestyle.

Patient B will have a negative set of beliefs around his back pain, expecting that he is doomed forever, that it can only get worse, that rest is the only cure, and that activity will cause more pain and therefore more damage. Because he's "been told by his doctor," he will now modify his behavior, become less active, develop more back pain because of his inactivity, and slowly spiral downwards into disability, chronic pain and dependency.

If over a period of time Patient B is repeatedly told by his doctor and other health professionals (nurses, therapists) that his back pain is due to degenerative disc disease, the message becomes reinforced and more entrenched in the patient's mind. And every time he modifies his behavior (does less) in response to the pain, he becomes more unfit and more prone to having back pain, reinforcing his own beliefs. These beliefs can also be inadvertently reinforced by loved ones and colleagues at work by being over concerned about the pain and telling them to do less, take it easy.

When the pain comes on with every movement, and the pain in the patient's mind means that his back has been damaged further, several things then happen:

- The patient becomes frightened to do anything that may cause the pain. This is called *Pain Avoidance Behavior* or fear of the pain.
- He anticipates the pain before he moves, causing him to hold his breath and guard his back, while tightening his back muscles. This is called *Guarded Movements*. Guarding only serves to increase the pain during movement, as most of the pain is muscular in the first place.
- Anxiety and depression develop over time with a tendency to exaggerate the pain, its cause, and its consequences (to make it seem worse than it actually is, to make the pain into a catastrophe). Anxiety and depression may also cause the patient to misinterpret the severity of the pain leading to a vicious spiral downwards.

When patient B eventually presents to a chronic pain clinic for help, he has firmly entrenched views about the pain, the cause, and how he should manage it. The clinic will examine his beliefs about the pain in order to try to help him, but the longer the abnormal beliefs have been held, the harder it is to change and the stronger the emotional reaction during the process of trying to change. The technical word for a belief is "cognition." Psychological treatment to try to re-educate the patient about his beliefs is called Cognitive Behavioral Therapy (CBT). Many chronic pain clinics have multidisciplinary teams (pain doctor, clinical psychologists and physiotherapists) who will try to use CBT to try to modify the patient's set of beliefs about the pain, in order for him to begin the long road towards physical and psychological rehabilitation. If the patient's beliefs cannot be changed, then he will not modify his behavior, and not win the battle against chronic pain. Some patients can manage their pain by combining CBT plus specialized physiotherapy, whereas others need some form of pain relieving procedure before embarking down this road. Whatever technique, the messages are the same:

- You must learn as much about your pain as possible through education.
- You must stop thinking that pain equals more damage.
- You must learn how to control the fear of the pain, and stop anticipating it by guarding your muscles.
- You have to stop obsessing about the pain, instead trying to minimize it in your mind, i.e., convince yourself it's only a muscle spasm.
- You must be as active as you possibly can be to prevent the negative consequences of inactivity.

In my line of work, I see many patients who are victims of MRI but no one as much as my thirty-eight year old patient, Brad. Before his illness, Brad owned and was skilled at operating heavy machinery—the kind of equipment that cost hundreds of thousands of dollars and employed workers year round. He was the son of German immigrants and at six-foot-four and 250 pounds, his employees paid attention to his orders, which always included a flash of his perfect white teeth. When I walked into the examining room on the day he came to see me, Brad was pacing back and forth. He stopped and extended a hand, smiling broadly. He said he was happy to finally see me.

I asked Brad why he was here and he pointed to a stack of MRI scans lying on the chair beside him. "I've been waiting to see you for weeks, Dr. Kachmann. I have horrible back pain and need surgery now." He began discussing every esoteric device used in the latest surgical techniques for back surgery. I could tell he had done his homework and then some.

Medical information online has pros and cons. One of the obvious pros is that it can prepare patients for appointments, help them research information and limit time on the phone with nurses and doctors. One of the downfalls is that, by nature of the medium, medical information can be oversimplified and misleading. Consumers may attempt to understand pathology by examining the tiniest pieces of it, and then extrapolate from those pieces to overarching surmises about the whole.

Chronic back pain often responds 30 to 100 percent from massage, Tai Chi and Qigong. Knowing that, surgery should not be the first choice for degenerative disc pain. Because conventional medicine is based on diseases that often have a single cause, mainstream physicians have, for the most part, failed to treat complex chronic pain illnesses. Medicare plays a key role in shaping patient's choices, too. The Medicare payment system rewards complexity, it lets doctors bill for the individual procedures they perform within a single surgery and encourages the development of advanced technologies. Many private insurers wait for the government's decision before setting their own coverage policies.

Nearly all back pain is caused by strains and sprains to the muscles and ligaments that support the spine. These soft-tissue injuries usually heal within six weeks or so. Most people may find pain relief in conservative treatments such as rest, physical therapy, anti-inflammatory medications or epidural injections. Many older people who experience chronic back pain are suffering from degenerative changes in the spine's structure, which happens to a varying degree in all of us. Imaging devices like CT and MRI offer detailed pictures of these kinds of problems but often don't reveal which changes explain the pain. Although back surgery is a cure for some, most people suffering from stress-related back pain will improve by following the mind-body therapies.

Additionally, surgery has risks and long recovery time. After spinal fusion surgery, restrictions on activities may last 6-12 months, the time your body needs to grow new bone between metal implants. Fusion can significantly reduce a patient's range of motion; sometimes, it can accelerate the deterioration of the discs above and below where the fusion took place, because the lumbar spine is meant to move. There are five segments in the spine. If you take one or two of those away, the motion has to be made up for by the remaining segments, which are going to be subject to increased stress compared to a normal spine. In many cases, pain returns after a couple years of respite and re-operation is necessary. In the end, you're fighting the normal changes of aging.

People are generally more satisfied with their outcome when they employ self-healing initiatives such as stress-reduction, weight-loss and exercise in lieu of surgery. When assessing a complaint of pain, doctors must also investigate the appropriate psychological and environmental factors. Pain is an experience and cannot be separated from the patient's mental state; a surgeon's hand cannot fix what within the patient's mind.

Would Brad really feel better after the surgery? Not for long, and in the end, he would incur thousands and thousands of dollars in medical bills.

"Sit down," I said. "Let's talk."

Brad lived in an upper class suburb of Indianapolis. He and his father owned one of the top ten asphalt companies in the US. His father had come to America as an infant after the Greek defeat of Italy in 1940. Despite the enormous superiority of the Italian forces, the Greek army forced the Italians into a massive retreat deep into Albania.

Brad had divorced his wife Katherine, with whom he had three children, when he was 36-years-old. The following year he embarked on a tempestuous one-year marriage to a marketing director at work. The union fell apart when Brad had an affair with another employee that resulted in a baby. In total, Brad fathered four children.

Because the family business provided everything from manufacturing asphalt to paving surfaces in four Midwestern states, Brad was constantly traveling. To cope with the stress of his job and alimony responsibilities, he said he smoked and drank five or six beers a night. Worse, he had become hooked on narcotics. Addiction is a complicated disorder affecting brain processes responsible for motivation, decision making, pleasure seeking, inhibitory control and the way we learn and consolidate information and experiences.

Brad wore a fentanyl patch for his back pain, a prescription-only product that is intended for cancer patients and others with chronic pain. The patch is designed to dispense medicine slowly through the skin, but at least seven deaths in Indiana, and four in South Carolina since 2005 have been blamed on abuse of the patch, along with more than 100 deaths in Florida in 2004.[171]

We know from many rigorous studies that social support networks, such as a happy marriage, satisfying job or involvement in a church, protect against disabling pain syndromes. It troubled Brad that he was dependent on pain medication, but he had made peace with the need for it. Like many people suffering from chronic pain, he had crossed the threshold of self-recovery and hope; his pain had become him.

As far as I could tell, Brad wanted to feel better and started taking painkillers for the same reasons that most people start taking them:

because they work. They're quick and easy to coax from practitioners' prescription pads. In turn, doctors troubled by the most difficult to treat patients welcome painkillers to keep patients like Brad pacified. Surgeons, especially, tend to be dismissive of nonphysical back pain, filing it away under the proverbial "psyche case" cabinet of the mind. Surgeons tend to think in mechanistic terms—removing the cause of pain by fusing the spine, pinning or casting the fracture, removing the appendix or clipping the aneurysm.

According to the Mayo Clinic, pain is the most common symptom that brings patients to a doctor's office, but it remains one of the least understood. There's no scan or blood test to objectively measure the level of a person's pain, and years of research have determined that different people experience pain very differently. The same helplessness and hopeless that can befriend organic disease often accompanies pain from unexplained symptoms, further limiting functional status and quality of life.[172] People with chronic pain tend to have lower than normal levels of painkilling endorphins and need to be taught techniques like visualization and meditation that can help trigger and perpetuate the body's own painkillers.

Pain and the Brain

Pain is the primary complaint that prompts people to see a doctor, sending far more women to pain clinics than men. Perhaps more than any other aspect of experience, persistent pain is something we cannot control. Therefore, we need to think about pain as the result of complex interfaces between the brain and our own capacity to regulate its severity and significance. A build up of chemicals like dopamine suppress the activity of the brain's natural painkillers. Self-healing techniques such as meditation, hypnosis and Tai Chi or yoga, all of which we'll discuss more in-depth in Part IV, can reduce or even block the perception of pain in your brain. In fact, your beliefs can shut-down the pain-modulatory system even when the wound is still open (the placebo effect). Similarly, your beliefs can increase pain if you believe you are being hurt, even if you aren't (the nocebo effect). Music, meditation or visualization and hypnosis can result in a reduction of rACC activation—the area of the brain involved in mediating the conscious perception of pain.[173]

Pain Clinics

Since 1973, the multidisciplinary pain clinic has come into its own. Many clinics now offer a variety of therapeutic approaches to effective pain management, including physical therapy, acupuncture, TENS (transcutaneous electronic nerve stimulation), hypnosis, and behavioral modification. However, not all patients have access to good pain clinics and, in the US, many pain therapies focus on those that are habituating and addicting.

Drugs have potencies that far exceed normal levels of endogenously generated pain relievers and the brain adapts to this excessive stimulation or inhibition by neuroadaptation. When the drugs are taken away, people feel unstable. Combine these facts with varying biological predispositions and propensities of individuals and you have the problems associated with dependency. The expectations or fears of individuals add measurably to the severity of the problems associated with drugs.

Pain is a private perception that arises in the conscious brain, typically in response to a harmful stimulus, but sometimes in the absence of a stimulus. The perception to the stimulus varies from person to person, and depends on the person's expectations and beliefs, genes, cognitive and emotional state—not just the stimulus itself. Focusing on a pill to elicit euphoria or treat addiction fails to address the primary cause of becoming and staying hooked: the epidemic of stressful, disconnected lives.

"Those things that hurt, instruct," Benjamin Franklin said. Perhaps patients who suffer from chronic pain need to dig deeper and look for new answers. It's no longer possible to divide the process of pain from the experience or perception of pain; it's time for new approaches for the treatment of pain. Pain centers say the "gold standard" in treating chronic pain is the patient's word. In truth, the gold standard in treating chronic pain is diagnosis. Habituating and addicting a patient with an unclear diagnosis is borderline criminal.

The government estimates that pain-related illness costs the American public more than $100 billion each year in health care, compensation and litigation expenses.[174] Pain has become a political problem, too. The majority of Social Security Disability benefits are based on chronic pain problems. The need for further research into pain mechanisms and control was recognized by the US Congress in

MBI Categories: Stress Index

Normal Stress Levels	<20
Probable Mild Stress-related Symptoms	20-25
Probable Moderate Stress-related Symptoms	25-30
Probable Severe Stress-related Symptoms	30 +

Possible Stress-related Disorders

Acne	Infertility
Allergies	Insomnia
Anger Disorders	Irritable Bladder
Anxiety Disorders	Irritable Bowel Syndrome
Asthma Flare-up	Joint Pain
Autoimmune Disease	Menopause Syndrome
Back Pain	Metabolic Syndrome
Cardiac Arrhythmia	Migraine
Certain Cancers	Multiple Sclerosis Flare-up
Chest Pain	Muscle Tension
Chrohn's Disease	Perimenopause Syndrome
Chronic Fatigue Syndrome	Post-Traumatic Stress Disorder
Chronic Pain	Psoriasis Flare-up
Cold Sores	Repetitive Stress Injuries
Colitis Flare-up	Rheumatoid Disorders
Common Cold	Sexual Disorders
Constipation	Skin Diseases
Coronary Spasm	Skin Rash
Depression	Sleep Disorders
Diarrhea	Stomach Cramps
Eating Disorders	Substance Abuse
Fatigue	Tension Myositis
Fibromyalgia	Thoracic Outlet Syndrome
Glucose Intolerance	TMJ
Headache	Ulcer Flare-up
Hypertension	Worried Well

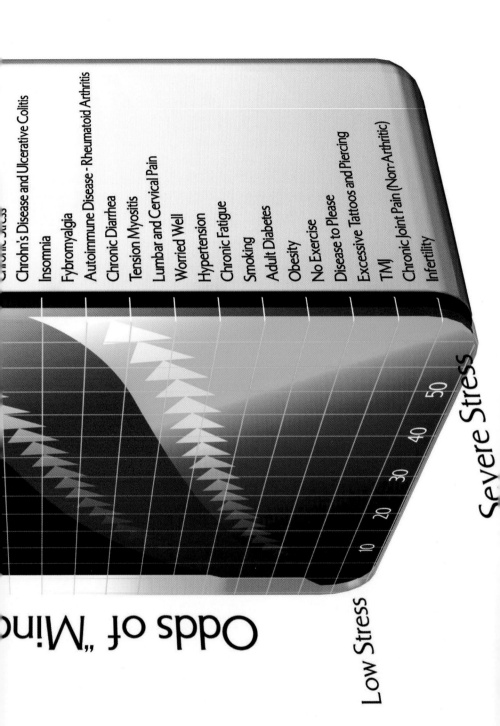

Odds of "Mind...

Chronic Stress
Chrohn's Disease and Ulcerative Colitis
Insomnia
Fybromyalgia
Autoimmune Disease - Rheumatoid Arthritis
Chronic Diarrhea
Tension Myositis
Lumbar and Cervical Pain
Worried Well
Hypertension
Chronic Fatigue
Smoking
Adult Diabetes
Obesity
No Exercise
Disease to Please
Excessive Tattoos and Piercing
TMJ
Chronic Joint Pain (Non-Arthritic)
Infertility

10   20   30   40   50

Severe Stress

Low Stress

MIND BODY INDEX

Stress Level
- Female
- Male

Irritable Bowel Syndrome
Back Pain
Chronic Pain
Depression Anger Fear
Headaches
Chronic Pelvic Pain and Bladder Spasm
Eating Disorders
Skin Diseases - Itching - 10 Diseases
Asthma
Chronic Chest Pain
Cardiac Arrhythmia
Esophageal Reflux (Gerd)
Chronic Constipation

d Body" Illness

Contemporary Stress [Put a check next to the stressors in your life]

■	Death of a spouse or child	10	■	Relationship problems	3
■	Death of a parent	9	■	Parent's divorce or remarriage	3
■	Divorce	7	■	Obesity	3
■	Acute serious illness	7	■	Poor living conditions	3
■	Depression	7	■	Long commute	3
■	Birth of a grandchild	6	■	Mortgage or loan over $30,000	3
■	Death of close family member	6	■	Major personal achievement	3
■	Caring for sick family member	6	■	History of childhood abuse	3
■	Personal injury	6	■	No exercise	3
■	Acute serious injury	6	■	Sleep disorder	3
■	Decreased income	6	■	Poor eating habits	3
■	Marital arguments	6	■	New residence	3
■	Fired from work	6	■	Change in work hours	3
■	Pregnancy	5	■	Change in work responsibilities	3
■	Miscarriage or abortion	5	■	Son or daughter leaving home	2
■	Chronic serious illness	5	■	Difficult in-law	2
■	Victim of crime	5	■	Difficult stepparent	2
■	Foreclosure on mortgage or loan	5	■	Change of school or college	2
■	Bankruptcy or investment crisis	5	■	Spouse begins or stops working	2
■	Jail term	5	■	Starting or finishing school	2
■	Divorced with young children	5	■	Technology overload	2
■	Death of a close friend	4	■	Trouble with boss	2
■	Retirement	4	■	Increased income	2
■	Caring for multiple young children	4	■	Watching television violence	2
■	Lack of job skills	4	■	Threat of terrorism or war	2
■	Lack of education	4	■	No recreational activities	2
■	Car or other accident	4	■	Loud noise	2
■	Change in family member's health	4	■	Contending with traffic	2
■	Addition to family	4	■	Minor law violation	2
■	Major life decision	4	■	Christmas season	2
■	Sexual difficulties	4	■	Change in political beliefs	2

Stress Index [Add together all of your stressors]

Column 1 [   ] + Column 2 [   ] = YOUR STRESS INDEX [   ] its declaration of the years 2001-2010 as the "Decade of Pain Control and Research."

Many pain centers have become "cash cows," businesses that generate profit margins so high that the profits far exceed the amount necessary to keep it going. As such, some pain clinics have become complacent, with management ignoring the need for change as market forces erode value, and negligent of clinical science, as the management in charge tries to garner support for their most profitable and "sticky" products—namely drugs and the demand of the addict. In my career as a neurosurgeon spanning almost 40 years, I've seen too many people over-treated with surgical procedures and addicted to painkillers.

When I scanned the hospital surgery schedule recently and saw at least twenty spine-injections (epidural blocks for pain), five days a week, I wondered, "Did anyone counsel the patient about breathing techniques, prayer, meditation or massage, visualization, or music therapy—all more holistic approaches that connect the mind, body and spirit?"

As stated earlier, the gold standard for assessing chronic pain is diagnosis, not the patient's word, which is contrary to the philosophy of most pain centers. I'm not suggesting that people in pain are "faking it," fabricating or exaggerating to gain powerful prescriptions (although some addicts will). The perceptual experience of pain, whether acute, chronic or any of the clinical types, is real. But treatment needs to involve an array of "mind-body" therapies. To write a prescription for narcotics because someone says, "I hurt," is completely inappropriate beyond a week or two unless the diagnosis is clear.

A patient recently joked that if a certain doctor at a local hospital left town, the entire city would go into withdrawal, a powerful observation which revealed the true state of medicine in America. We have become complacent. Too dependent on quick fixes, and happy that those quick fixes keep people quiet and line our pocketbooks.

Pain clinics will quote numerous pain studies that document the effects of different narcotics, tranquilizers or muscle relaxants, but they rarely discuss holistic therapies. My greatest concern is the rate of misdiagnosis by pain centers that choose to ignore mind-body factors. Unfortunately, non-prescription, non-procedural treatments just don't pay well.

To truly help the patient, the holistic approach should come first, not last. The goal of pain-relieving techniques such as meditation and hypnosis is to turn off nerve-firing that causes the perception of pain in the brain, as well as reduce the anxiety and psychological suffering that can accompany chronic pain.

When I was operating recently, I mentioned to an anesthesiologist that my daughter and I were writing a book on mind-body illness and treatment, including chronic pain syndromes. He said that last week he was working with a pain specialist who was injecting the spine (epidural block) of a 110 pound, eight-month-pregnant woman, not for labor and delivery, but for a backache. When he mentioned that the mother had the same treatment the week before, the whole operating room became quiet. As a patient, you may assume that if a doctor prescribes a medication, it's safe. But that's not always the case.

The treatment of pain has come a long way since inhaling ether, but how are we measuring progress? To consider the patient's word as the gold standard for pain treatment is like clipping the wires to your fire alarm when the house is burning and going back to sleep. The gold standard is proper diagnosis, psychological and stress evaluation and behavioral change, not pain relief with narcotics for weeks on end. One of the primary goals of this book is to motivate patients and health care providers to open their eyes and minds and raise their voices: habituating and addicting, over-treating stress-related pain and illness is not only killing the patient, but also killing the economy and ultimately, the medical community.

CHAPTER 9

Heart, a Mind of Its Own

Neither a lofty degree of intelligence nor imagination nor both together go to the making of genius. Love, love, love, that is the soul of genius.
— Wolfgang Amadeus Mozart

The writer John Gregory Dunne died of a heart attack at the end of 2003. His death came suddenly, just as he and his wife Joan were sitting down to dinner after visiting their daughter in the Intensive Care Unit, who was being treated for pneumonia and septic shock. Joan Didion wrote about the year of grieving after her husband's death in *The Year of Magical Thinking*. She quotes a study where "research to date has shown that, like many other stressors, grief frequently leads to changes in the endocrine, immune, autonomic nervous, and cardiovascular systems; all of these are fundamentally influenced by brain function and [biochemicals]."[175] Recent studies have determined that the "widower effect"—the chances a survivor will die after a spouse's death—is real. The burden of giving care or stress from a spouse's death could cause a withdrawal from social networks and an increase in unhealthy behavior, such as drinking, cessation of exercise, and eating unhealthy foods.

I opened the *New York Times* recently and read the headlines, "Enron Founder Dies Before Sentencing." The story said:

Kenneth Lay, who was convicted of fraud and conspiracy, faced the possibility of spending the rest of his life in prison. The financial crimes that Mr. Lay and Jeffrey K. Skilling, who succeeded Mr. Lay as chief executive and presided over Enron during its implosion, were convicted of committing came to symbolize the corporate excess and greed of the 1990's.[176]

And in March of 2006, I read in the *Times*, "Slobodan Milosevic, 64, Former Yugoslav Leader Accused of War Crimes, Dies." The story read:

Authorities with the U.N. war crimes tribunal are investigating the death of Slobodan Milosevic after the former Yugoslav president was found dead Saturday morning in his cell in The Hague, Netherlands. He was 64. Milosevic's death came just a few months before the expected conclusion of his trial, which had lasted more than four years. Autopsies soon established that Milosevic had died of a heart attack.[177]

While the brain is a complex biological organ of great computational capability that constructs our sensory experiences, regulates our thoughts and emotions, and controls our actions, these two examples show that the heart also serves as an information-processing center. The heart has a complex nervous system. On a more clinical level, we know that specialized neural circuits made up of nerve cells and neurotransmitters exist in different heart regions. Within these circuits, molecular substances generate signals within and between nerve cells (like the brain) to do what needs to be done at that moment. Nerve cells respond to these chemical signals that produce coordinated changes in heart rate independent of the brain. In other words, "Your heart has its own mind."[178]

Most cardiac deaths occur when electrical impulses in a diseased heart become rapid (ventricular tachycardia) or chaotic (ventricular fibrillation) or both. This irregular heart rhythm (arrhythmia) causes the heart to suddenly stop beating. When someone is agitated or afraid, the body's stress response kicks in, and prompts a rapid heartbeat, trembling and sweating. Adrenaline released during intense emotional states often act as a trigger for sudden death when abnormalities such as hypertension, heart disease or cardiomyopathy are present. Associations between emotional states and difficulties with the heart's electrical system have been cited in numerous scientific studies.

The September 11 terrorist attacks may have affected the heart, suggest studies from Yale and Columbia universities. Implantable cardioverter defibrillators (ICDs) likely prevented even more deaths in

Brain and Heart Communication

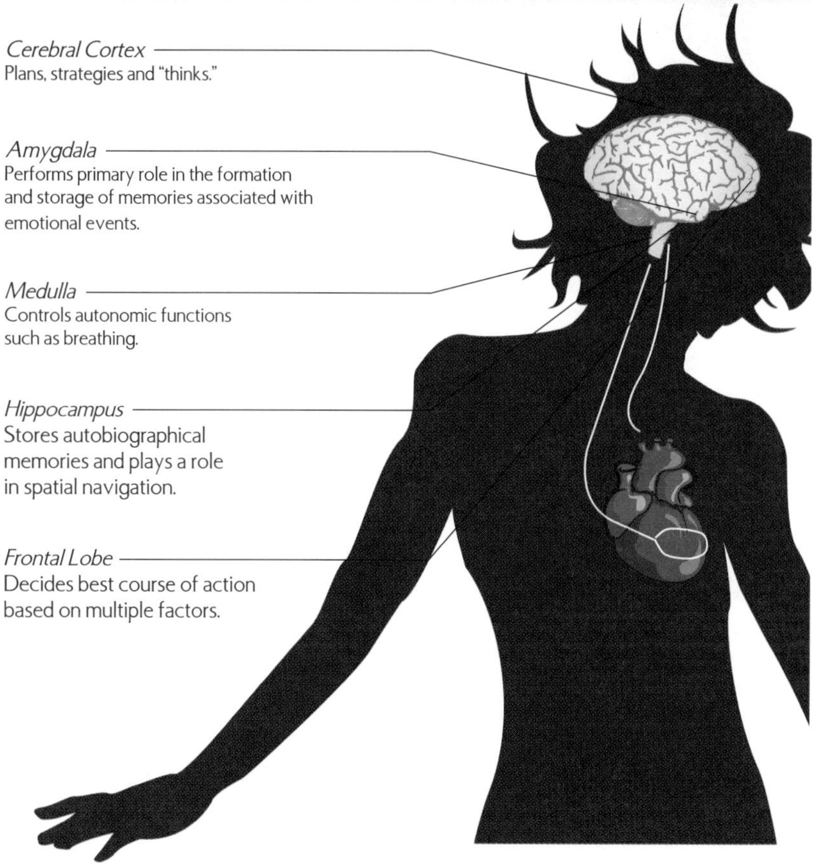

Cerebral Cortex
Plans, strategies and "thinks."

Amygdala
Performs primary role in the formation
and storage of memories associated with
emotional events.

Medulla
Controls autonomic functions
such as breathing.

Hippocampus
Stores autobiographical
memories and plays a role
in spatial navigation.

Frontal Lobe
Decides best course of action
based on multiple factors.

Figure 10: Two-way communication exists between the heart and brain to regulate heart rate and blood pressure. The interaction of signaling molecules flowing between the two organs causes the heart rate to vary with each beat. Your thoughts, perceptions and emotional reactions are transmitted from the brain to the heart via the sympathetic and parasympathetic nervous systems, and can be seen in the patterns of your heart rhythms on an EKG.

the wake of the tragedy: life-threatening rhythm disturbances increased more than two-fold in a group of ICD recipients in the month after the attacks, according to one study. ICDs are used in heart patients at risk for recurrent, sustained ventricular tachycardia or fibrillation. The device is connected to leads positioned inside the heart or on its surface. These leads are used to deliver electrical shocks, sense the cardiac rhythm and sometimes pace the heart, as needed.

Intense emotion caused by sports events like the Super Bowl or World Cup can lead to cardiac arrest, which not only happens to fans with cardiovascular disease but also to some healthy fans. Eleven soccer fans died of cardiac arrest in China during the 2006 World Cup. Chinese officials called the incidents a part of a "World Cup Syndrome." Previous studies have shown that sporting fervor can lead to anxiety, panic and even heart attacks in some fans.

Scientists studied stress in World Cup Soccer fans with the help of volunteers who measured the heart rate of the volunteers every five seconds. A computer then averaged the readings over each minute. Additionally, saliva volumes and composition were measured and there were questionnaire responses. During the first experiment at the England-Paraguay game some fans' heart rates rose to 95-100 beats per minute (BPM) compared with the normal 70 BPM. The researchers also measured the amount of cortisol, a stress hormone related to adrenaline, in the saliva. Volunteers in the study at the soccer game produced on average *half* the usual amount of saliva, pointing to higher stress levels that tend to dry out the mouth.

The prestigious medical journal *Circulation* published a study which concluded that reducing emotional distress through a rehabilitation program improved the prognosis of people with heart disease. Social isolation, depression and anxiety strongly correlate with a person's prognosis. Emotional states not only contribute to heart disease and coronary events, but even pose a greater risk than second-hand smoke.

Perhaps most alarming of all, life-threatening heart arrhythmias occur more often at the beginning or end of the work week. Workers who are under constant stress may start to show it in their blood pressure readings. In a study that followed more than 6,719 white-collar workers for 7.5 years, Canadian researchers found that those with high job demands, and reported low levels of social support in the office, tended to have higher blood pressure than other workers.[179] Prominent studies suggest that negative emotions may trigger cardiovascular events during the anticipation or preparation of a stressful event.

Stress can even "break" your heart. "Broken heart syndrome" is a rare cardiac disorder that mimics a heart attack. Some people, especially women, may respond to sudden, overwhelming emotional stress such as a such as the death of a loved one, car accident or even the intense emotional stress of a wedding by releasing large amounts of adrenaline, cortisol and other potent chemicals into the blood stream. These chemicals can be temporarily toxic to the heart, effectively stunning the muscle and producing symptoms similar to a heart attack or heart failure: chest discomfort, sweating, shortness of breath and swelling. The condition is fatal in some individuals and results in life-threatening complications in others. However, most people who suffer from broken heart syndrome regain full cardiac function.

My Daughter's Heart

As we discussed in the chapter on placebo or nocebo, each interaction between a doctor and a patient is an opportunity to make a difference. A negative experience with a health care provider can be harmful and even cause "nocebo effects" with varying degrees of harm. My family experienced nocebo effects firsthand.

During my daughter's third pregnancy, she began experiencing irregular heart beats for the first time in her life, and finally went to see a local cardiologist who reassured her that the palpitations were normal for pregnancy. Five months into the pregnancy, they worsened, however, and she began experiencing an unprecedented "squeezing" chest and neck pressure. She also had trouble breathing and felt like she was wearing lead boots. The change in her health and stamina were dramatic. She had worked full time during her fist two pregnancies, and even jogged three miles several times a week. Like many people confronting the unknown, my daughter sought second and third medical opinions about her symptoms.

Her second cardiologist listened to her heart with a stethoscope while leaning forward—something her first cardiologist didn't do. He also said her condition wasn't "benign" or simply due to the pregnancy. He requested an echocardiogram the next day, which revealed three heart valves leaking—rare for someone her age and gender, and signs that her heart *could be* abnormally enlarging. The extra demands on the heart from pregnancy typically don't enlarge the heart to a pathological degree.

Pregnancy-induced changes in the cardiovascular system develop primarily to meet the increased metabolic demands of the mother and baby. Despite the increased workload of the heart during gestation and labor, most women have no impairment of cardiac reserve. Blood volume increases progressively from 6-8 weeks gestation during pregnancy, and reaches a maximum volume at approximately 32-34 weeks. The extra demands on my daughter's heart in combination with an elusive condition called "microvascular disease" were causing her symptoms. But for months, we had no idea what the cause was.

Soon after her echocardiogram, my daughter developed superficial venous thrombophlebitis (SVT)—a benign blood clot in comparison to deep vein thrombosis (DVT) that can travel to the lungs. Instead of saying that SVT was superficial and benign, her doctor told her that it was a serious disorder, warning her that the blood clot could travel. He prescribed bed rest. This was the same week in 2003 that a CNN reporter died suddenly in Iraq from a pulmonary embolism. My daughter started to show signs of anxiety.

For the next four months of her pregnancy, my daughter kept her leg elevated, used warm compresses and wore support hose during the stifling summer heat. She also drafted her first *Living Will and Last Testament*, studied vascular disease and learned to recognize the symptoms of pulmonary embolism and heart attack.

Two days before the end of her pregnancy, she called her doctor to once again describe the mysterious rising, constricting pressure that traveled from the middle of her chest into her neck and jaw. Unlike labor pains, the pressure traveled into her chest instead of her belly and legs. Her doctor told her that her symptoms were anxiety-related: "Valve regurgitation doesn't cause chest pain—only big, bad heart disease does," he said. After hearing about her doctor's dismissive response to a potentially life-threatening symptom, I decided to get on the next plane.

The day I arrived, my daughter went into labor and I offered to call an ambulance. Her husband insisted to drive her and asked that I remain at home on "stand by." Her contractions were a minute-and-a-half apart.

Two hours after her admittance to the hospital, the anesthesiologist (whom she described as the nefarious "Romano" on TV's ER) read her medical history and asked if she had had an angiogram. He also asked the nurse for her vitals. The nurse said she had forgotten to take them. Earning his namesake, "Romano" cursed the nurse and asked my daughter how she was feeling. "I feel cold and my chest is tight," her husband recalled.

Romano went into full crisis mode, triggering a "Code Blue" in the Labor and Delivery room. My son-in-law called me on my cell phone and asked for my advice. I said that I would be right over.

When I arrived at my daughter's hospital room, I asked for her chart and read that her blood pressure had dropped to 55/35 even before the epidural (anesthesia), and "Romano" had administered ephedrine (adrenaline) to stimulate her heart. More than shock or sadness, I felt anger. At this critical moment in my relationship with my daughter, I realized that her symptoms, as rare and unbelievable as they are for someone her age, were real. I vowed to help her in any way that I could as a doctor, father and grandfather.

As if the data in her chart weren't bad enough, I also learned that right before my daughter had fainted, the nurse had asked for her Living Will and whether she was an organ donor. When she came to, her nurse apologized, saying, "Your lips had turned white."

Why anyone, especially a trained health care professional, would ask such a question during a dire life or death moment is beyond me, and to this day it makes me shake. There was something perverted about this scene: a young woman losing consciousness, dropping to the floor, possibly never waking up, and the last words she hears are *whether or not she was an organ donor?* How would you feel if instead of a healing prayer, compassionate or loving words upon your death you heard that bone-chilling question repeated a million times at the state licensing bureau, "Are you an organ donor?"

Has American medicine come to that? Do we consider a thinking, feeling, living, breathing human life is an accumulation of body parts?

By the grace of God (and under the care of an alert, take-no-prisoners anesthesiologist), my daughter delivered a seven-pound boy at 3:30am on July 23, 2003. The moral to this story is that early detection, accurate diagnosis and proper treatment of heart disease can save a life, sometimes two.

The morning after the drama of labor and delivery, Kim's obstetrician sat down beside her bed and said, "What you have can kill you. It can kill you." That night my daughter woke from a nightmare. Her doctor had given her the ultimate nocebo. Research suggests that women who believe they are prone to heart disease are nearly four times as likely to die as women with similar risk factors who didn't hold such fatalistic views. "They're convinced that something is going to go wrong, and it's a self-fulfilling prophecy," said Arthur Barsky in the

Washington Post.[180] Barsky is a psychiatrist at Boston's Brigham and Women's Hospital who published his study on women in JAMA and like me, implores his peers to pay closer attention to the nocebo effect. As a doctor, nurse, assistant or technician, you are the patient's health care experience, and as such, your word has a powerful effect on healing.

Heart Disease in America

Cardiovascular disease accounts for 29.2 percent of total global deaths, according to the World Health Organization (WHO). About 20 million people survive heart attack and stroke each year, but many require long-term treatment. Coronary heart disease is usually the clinical manifestation of an underlying pathological process called "atherosclerosis." The progression of atherosclerosis usually leads to narrowing of the arteries and eventually coronary flow deficits, resulting in cardiac electrical instability, heart attack and or heart failure. Cardiac arrest occurs when the heart suddenly stops working, most commonly due to a heart-rhythm disturbance called ventricular fibrillation (VF). In VF, the electrical impulses controlling the heartbeat become chaotic, causing the ventricles—the heart's main pumping chambers—to quiver instead of contracting as they should. Unless VF is corrected by an electrical shock from a defibrillator device or machine, the person can die within minutes.

To complicate matters, the symptoms of heart disease differ in men and women. Men typically experience angina—chest pain or squeezing pressure in the middle of the chest, sometimes extending to the left arm. Women, like my daughter, can experience nausea, shortness of breath and discomfort in the left jaw, arm or underneath the left breast or even in the back. Until recently, doctors thought men were more prone to heart disease but research and population studies indicate that it affects men and women equally, although women tend to experience it later in life. Women also tend to experience microvascular heart disease, a "hidden" disease where plaque builds in the smaller arterioles leading from the larger arteries in the heart, which puts them at risk for the same complications as "big, bad" heart disease: heart attack, heart failure and stroke.

Epidemiological and experimental studies showing the cause of coronary heart disease have progressed over the past few decades. Many studies now link stress and intense emotional states to blood pressure, elevated lipid concentrations and unhealthy behavioral patterns like smoking and anger to eruption of plaques within the walls of arteries, creating a cascade of events leading to myocardial infarction (heart attack) or lethal arrhythmias.

Injury to the inner lining of the artery or "endothelial dysfunction" from smoking, prediabetes or genetics initiates the disease and can lead to vasospasms, ischemia (lack of blood flow) and arrhythmia or sudden cardiac death. A progressive plaque may interfere with the ability of the artery wall (endothelial lining) to widen in response to the body's hemodynamic demands.

Traditional risk factors such as diabetes, smoking and hypertension are not the only risk factors for cardiovascular disease. Mounting evidence suggests that your psychological outlook and social networks are critical. Our intuition has progressed to a search for the scientific mechanisms underlying cardiovascular events related to emotion. In a recent study, people feeling loved or supported by friends and family had lower rates of coronary occlusion than unsupported subjects. The effects of stress on the autonomic nervous system, which controls, among other vital processes, the working of the heart, may explain the connection between emotions and heart health.

Many studies have examined the link between cardiovascular disease and job strain, typically defined as work with high psychological demands but with little independence or decision-making authority. Jobs such as assembly-line worker, garment worker, waiter and cook have high demands and low control and were found to have much higher rates of heart attack than white collar managerial jobs. Stress might raise blood pressure by chronically activating the nervous and cardiovascular systems. On the other hand, stressed workers may have little time or energy for exercise, may eat poorly or may have higher smoking rates.[181]

"Inflammation" is the process by which the body responds to injury, and as we have discussed in the chapter on pain, the triggers for inflammation are complex and involve immune system to brain communication systems. Research suggests that inflammation is an important mechanism in atherosclerosis or heart disease. This is the process in which fatty deposits build up in the lining of arteries. Immune cells living in plaques make prostaglandins, key players in inflammation that make the plaques more vulnerable to rupture. Recently, geneticists fingered the first common gene associated with inflammation and a higher risk of both heart attacks and strokes. Leukotrienes, which contribute to asthma in part by constricting airways, may play a central role in cardiovascular disease. But genetic predisposition is only part of the reason why people develop heart disease—environmental factors play an even larger role.

Prevention, Not Plumbing

While we all come into the world with genetic predispositions, we must learn behaviors that contribute to sickness or health. In a series of studies about the impact of lifestyle changes and cardiovascular disease, Dean Ornish, M.D. found a strong correlation between adherence and outcome: the more his patients changed their life-style and diet by eating low-fat foods, exercising and training their minds to relax, the more improvements were noted on their imaging scans and angiograms. Age and degree of illness weren't the driving factors in reversing heart disease. Ornish proved the mind-body connection extends to the heart. He recommends daily stress management techniques, including diet, yoga stretching, breathing exercises, meditation and imagery and support groups. Study after study now shows that people who feel lonely and depressed are more likely to get sick and die prematurely than those who have a strong connection and a caring community.[182]

Walking 20 or 30 minutes a day at a comfortable pace can reduce premature death by 50 percent or more in people with known heart disease. Exercise helps to reverse the abnormal heart patterns that appear in patients after experiencing heart failure by suppressing certain neurohormones that cause many of the severe symptoms. In addition to exercise, breathing techniques are a safe intervention that can help patients with chronic heart failure, particularly those with weakness in breathing muscles.

Fish oil supplements provide omega-3 fatty acids that are protective to the heart and have other significant benefits such as reducing inflammation. And conventional medicines such as cholesterol-lowering drugs can be beneficial. They cause your liver to produce less cholesterol, which reduces both the likelihood of blockages building up in arteries as well as inflammation. Try making diet changes before starting on medication.

Critics blame cheap and easily available food for making us fat and escalating the rate of heart disease in Americans. A plethora of fast food restaurants and the mighty power of marketing super-sizes influence poor food choices. Food expert Brian Wansink, Ph.D. said in his book, *Mindless Eating*: "No one goes to bed skinny and wakes up fat. Most people gain (or lose) weight so gradually they can't really figure out how it happened."[183] Wansink recommends eating 20 percent less than you think you might want before you start to eat. Trimming 100-200 calories a day can make you 10 pounds lighter in 10 months, a sustainable goal. Diets low in fat may be enough to prevent heart disease in some, but it's not sufficient to reverse it in most people. Recent studies indicate that the Mediterranean-style diets, rich in healthy fats from olive oil or walnuts, may be better for the heart than low-fat regimens.

When you look at the risk factors for heart disease—high blood pressure, bad cholesterol and inflammation—stress hormones only make them worse. Stress hormones protect us in dangerous situations or when we have to perform. We produce sugar for energy. Our blood vessels constrict and platelets become stickier during an injury so we don't bleed to death. But what happens when we're bombarded all day long with situations that we *perceive* as stressful?

Two people can be in the same room, facing the same situation but may perceive it differently. "We boil at different degrees," said philosopher Ralph Waldo Emerson. One person may experience the stress response described by Walter Cannon. The other person may focus and use the relaxation response pioneered by Herbert Benson. If the brain perceives something as stressful, the adrenal glands produce cortisol to raise blood sugar and fuel the muscles. The kidneys produce aldosterone, a steroid hormone that raises blood pressure, furthering preparing the body for action. Stress will also trigger the body to produce adrenaline and noradrenalin, which raises cholesterol, constricts blood vessels and increases heart rate, all of which may cause skipped heartbeats, chest pain and that anxious feeling of apprehension. Adrenaline is even known to make platelets stickier.

Stress isn't the only emotion with the potential to do harm. The Greek word meaning "constriction" is the root of "anger" and "angina." Recent studies suggest that hostility may be more predictive of coronary disease than traditional factors, such as smoking. Anger and hostility also trigger the production of immune proteins involved in inflammation called IL-6, which may contribute to arterial thickening.[185] In people who are prone to anger, hostility or revenge, studies using heart rate monitors have shown that their heart rate variability (HRV) is in sympathetic overload. And in that constantly stimulated state, people are more prone to constricted arteries, high blood pressure and heart attack or stroke. *Anger kills.* Redford Williams, M.D. and Virginia Williams, Ph.D. wrote a best-selling book with the same name. They offer 17 practical strategies to overcome hostile, cynical or aggressive behaviors. Depression is especially hard on the cardiovascular system.

About 10 percent of the US adult population suffers from a depressive disorder.[185] Depressed people are more likely to smoke, overeat or drink too much alcohol and less likely to keep active, promoting obesity and perpetuating depression. Cardiac rehabilitation patients who have symptoms of depression take longer to return to their normal heart rate after taking a treadmill stress test. Heart rate recovery after exercise is an indication of how well the autonomic nervous system functions. Patients who take longer to recover their normal heart rate have an increased risk of mortality.[186]

Fortunately, anger disorders and depression are treatable with psychotherapy, group therapy, medications, or getting up and getting out for a walk. Depression, like any form of pain, is a sign that we need to change the way we're doing something, transforming our lives for the better. Regulating emotional states is as important as monitoring cholesterol, blood pressure and sugar levels.

The Wisdom of the Heart

The heart beats on average 72 BPM, or more than 100,000 beats a day. Why is the Waltz so relaxing? Both the heart and the Waltz move in the rhythm of three-quarter time. Heart rate, blood pressure and breathing rate fluctuate in response to music. Music can induce relaxation and reduce sympathetic activity. Music may even make us smarter. Listening to music while exercising increased scores on a verbal fluency test among cardiac rehabilitation patients, according the journal *Heart & Lung*. "Listening to music may influence cognitive function through different pathways in the brain. The combination of music and exercise may stimulate and increase cognitive arousal while helping to organize cognitive output."[187]

The FDA recently approved a Walkman-type device, called "Resperate" to lower blood pressure by playing alternating tones that help regulate breathing rates. A sensor strapped to the chest monitors inhalations and exhalations and uses the data to adjust the intervals between the tones, one that prompts a user to breathe in and the other to breathe out. The goal is for the patient to perform 10 breaths per minute and make relaxing breathing patterns a habit. A study in the *Journal of Clinical Hypertension* found that using the device for at least 15 minutes daily reduced systolic blood pressure (the force with which blood is pumped out of the heart) enough to lower some users' need for medication.

The heart is more than a ten-ounce pump, transporting oxygenated blood to the brain and other organs. Aristotle thought it was the seat of the soul. In her fascinating book *The Heart Speaks*, Mimi Guarnneri, M.D. says:

> The electromagnetic current of the heart is sixty times higher in amplitude than the field of the brain. It also emits an energy field five thousand times strong than the brain's, one that can be measured more than ten feet from the body.[188]

Literature, art and music have been made about the romantic qualities of the heart. Love is a feeling that people relate to the heart. We know that fear is generated by the amygdala in the limbic system, but the limbic system only functions properly when a person feels love and connection.[189] "If a new medication had the same impact, failure to prescribe it would be malpractice."[190] The body is the temple of the Holy Spirit in the Bible; the heart is the proverbial seat of the soul in all religions. I always pray with my patients before surgery—spiritual connections are powerful. Prayers are expressions of empathy that strengthen a caring community and bring comfort to those who are suffering. Comfort in this context undoubtedly has therapeutic health benefits. "The human body experiences a powerful gravitational pull in the direction of hope. That is why the patient's hopes are the physician's secret weapon. They are the hidden ingredients in any prescription," said Norman Cousins in his book, *Anatomy of an Illness*.

The anonymity and loss of community in our society are key factors in the rise of heart disease. The heart is nourished by relationships with other people; studies show that loneliness and isolation are risk factors. Social and cultural factors have powerful effects on cardiovascular functioning. Even owning a dog can help keep your blood pressure in check. The old adage that "money can't bring you happiness" is true, but it's even truer for people facing heart disease. All the stents and bypass technologies in the world can't buy you lasting heart health.

In my position as a neurosurgeon, I have spent years learning to have an open mind and even longer striving to have an open heart. Today when I examine patients, I try to look into their heart as much as their minds to help them heal. Guarneri comments on the state of cardiovascular medicine today, which mirrors my sentiments about the state of neurosurgery and medicine in general when she said, "I began to have a series of unfolding realizations. One was an awareness that my medical practice was making me less a doctor than a high-tech plumber, trained to sit and wait for someone to have a heart attack than to prevent one from happening."[191] Americans spend $18 billion annually on heart disease with an average $50,000 for open-heart surgery, or $10,000 for an angiogram. If we followed a more thoughtful approach to medical care, we could avoid over-treatment and help prevent heart disease. As Ornish would say, surgery bypasses the problem. "It's a little like mopping the floor under a leaky sink without turning off the faucet. Sometimes you have to mop the floor, but if you don't turn off the faucet, the problem comes back again."[192]

CHAPTER 10

Gut, a Hidden Brain

Emotions that have no vent in tears make the organs weepy.

–Verdi

On New Year's Eve a few years ago, I received a call that a colleague's wife, Julia, had arrived in the Emergency Room after a series of worsening headaches and seizures. Her husband Charles was a well-known cardiologist and president of the hospital board who referred several cases to my neurological group throughout the year. Julia was a popular French teacher at my children's school known for her compassion and unconventional creativity. She often wore long flowing fringe-covered skirts and a raspberry beret, playing the character of a beatnik artist. To break up the monotony of the conventional teaching routine, she would stand on her desk and recite French poems or write benign curse words in French on the chalkboard, covering them with her back and softly berating the children to recall their vocabulary words, or else she would call the principal and reveal the words on the chalkboard, pinning the blame on the lazy student. Her family lived down the street in a three-story stucco home with a green-tiled roof and pretty gardens. Their children Catherine, Charlie and Henry were in elementary and middle school with my four children.

When I arrived at Julia's dim-lit room in the ICU of the hospital on the southwest side of town, she greeted me with a glint of a smile in her eyes. I could tell she was in pain but she didn't complain. Charlie and Henry were tucked under her arms, and almost two-year-old Cathy was sucking her thumb on her mother's lap. I will never forget the sight of her children draped around her full body, as if they could shield their beloved mother from harm. Julia seemed calm. Her blood pressure was 180/90, her respirations were even but rapid, and her pupils were equal and reactive. An EEG (brain wave test) and angiographic scan revealed a bulging posterior communicating artery, a 1.5 cm blood clot in the small branch off the carotid artery. Her medical history was insignificant—no head injury, vascular disease, smoking or hypertension. While intracranial aneurysms are common, the blood clot was a medical mystery in an otherwise healthy middle-age woman. I recommended that we wait until the morning to operate.

I perform approximately 400 operations a year but unlike laminectomies and other routine back and brain surgeries, clipping aneurysms are never routine. The rate of complication without surgery is about 50 percent, including the possibility of a cerebral hematoma (brain bleed); ventricular rupture (brain rupture); hydrocephalus (brain edema); vasospasm and infarction (stroke or heart attack); and herniation (brain shifts). To top it off, in any patient with an aneurysm, there's a 15 – 20 percent chance of finding multiple aneurysms. The mortality rate and major morbidity risk is about 3.5 percent for aneurysm surgery performed by a skilled physician. Most people would benefit from surgery.

Once a decision is made to take an aneurysm to the table, I typically wrap up my day at the office, eat a high protein dinner and play a game of singles. I've discovered that the repetitive motions of tennis are a diversion from the day-to-day demands of life-and-death decision-making of neurosurgery. Tennis imposes and restores order. The game also gives me the sense of mastery I need in order to do what I have to do: cut into soft flesh, drill into the hard bone of the cranium, and manipulate brain tissue with the consistency of tofu. I also try to go to bed early.

That night, I lay awake for hours with the image of Julia's young children on her hospital bed and lap, cleaving to her bosom and shunning my arrival as if I were responsible for their mother's illness. I tried to focus and employ the visualization techniques I knew well by going over the surgery again and again in my mind's eye … but I couldn't sleep. So I went downstairs into the kitchen, cut a piece or two of perfumed-smelling peach pie and turned on the television before going back to bed.

Around 3:00am, I woke with a rumbling in my gut. Psychological factors are known to play a significant role in many gastric and intestinal (GI) processes, and I'm not immune to them. The sympathetic nervous system triggers the effect; the stress hormone acetylcholine excites the parasympathetic system, which in turn accelerates GI function. Symptoms include a variety of fluid eruptions, including increased saliva, vomiting, belching or diarrhea.

While I was chief resident of neurosurgery at Georgetown University Medical Center, I mentored a medical student who vomited every time he saw blood, causing substantial embarrassment for himself and confusion and delays in the surgical routine. Once when I was tapping a small mallet against a chisel into the base of the skull bone, blood spurted out like a fountain from a large subdural hematoma (blood clot) on the brain. The young medical student barely had time to turn away and vomit on the sanitized floors of the surgical theater. We left the surgery for precious minutes. I sent him for psychiatric counseling afterwards. He eventually overcame his affliction, (although his path towards recovery wasn't an elegant one). Stress affects everyone differently. Other stress-related GI symptoms may include heartburn, stomach cramps, nausea, and constipation. Loss of appetite can also sometimes be a result of stress. Others might eat more when stressed, and gain weight.

Needless-to-say, your gut has a mind of its own. Nerve cells in the gut act as an independent brain. Neurogastroenterologists theorize that we have one brain at the top of the spinal cord, another in the center of the chest (the heart) and a powerful third concealed in the gut, known as the enteric nervous system (ENS). Neurogastroenterology is a research area in the field of gastroenterology advanced by Michael Gershon, M.D. who refers to the interactions between the nervous and digestive systems as the "brain-gut axis." The field of neurogastroenterology began when scientists discovered that the gut contains a neuroplexus-neurotransmitter system that, like the heart, can operate without the brain.[193]

The vagus nerve, which sits in the medulla or center of the brain stem, is the conduit for messenger molecules traveling between the nervous and digestive systems. Like all of the organs in your body, the biochemical substrates of thought and emotion—hormones, neurotransmitters and peptides—can signal the digestive system and visa versa. Food and drink can elicit emotional states by triggering these chemicals through various glands, and certain thoughts and feelings can trigger gastric secretions in the stomach and intestines. The gut is another key component of the body's psychosomatic mind-body network.

The gut is a tube that has a lumen (cavity) end to end with a lining like our skin but more complex. The surface of the bowel must protect us from bacteria and excessive loss of water. Absorption means the transportation of digested nutrients and waste products across the lining of the bowel to reach the blood and lymph vessels in the wall of the intestine. Digestion and absorption are as important to life as a beating heart. The stomach has its own digestive enzymes, including pepsin which breaks down proteins. Pepsin has to work in acid, hydrochloric acid which is made by the stomach. As you know, this is nasty stuff and the stomach makes it very strong. Iron would dissolve in this acid but the lining of the stomach is tough. Acid can't dissolve it. Your esophagus isn't as strong, as people who experience heartburn or dyspepsia, or esophageal reflux can tell you from firsthand experience.

The autonomic nervous system has great influence on the stomach, bowel, and intestine, slowing down digestion during the fight-or-flight response. Communication between the brain, gut and immune system is also constant and has self-healing and self-monitoring components. The bowel's ENS connects to blood vessels and muscles and has about 100 million nerve cells but only a few thousand pre-ganglia (connections to the nervous system and brain) which are why some scientists refer to the gut as a second brain. The brain can cause pancreatic secretions, as well as the gut itself through hormones coming in from the blood. The brain delivers messages through the vagus nerve and sympathetic nervous system. The pancreas secrets important enzymes for digestion and insulin for blood sugar metabolism.

The ENS contains all of the biochemicals of emotion—neurotransmitters, neuropeptides and hormones. Nerves speak with a chemical language, but the molecular receptors in the smooth muscle of bowel and blood vessels must be receptive to the binding agent. When receptors from the ligand-receptor system in the gut are studied with radioisotopes, the bowel lights up like a Christmas tree. Gershon proved serotonin is made largely in the bowel, not the brain as previously thought. The chemistry behind the gut can explain why our bowels and stomachs sometimes react to depression or stress in "ungraceful" ways and may develop hiccups (no pun intended) in the system which creates functional disorders such as irritable bowel syndrome.

Irritable bowel syndrome (IBS) is an often painful and life-altering disorder that affects an estimated 30 million Americans, or 10-15 percent of the US population and more often women than men.[194] IBS is characterized by recurrent or persistent abdominal pain associated with altered stool frequency or consistency, and represents the most common reason for an individual to visit a gastroenterologist or primary care physician. Abnormalities in smooth muscle tone in the gastrointestinal tract during stress in patients with irritable bowel syndrome may contribute to symptoms. Medicine has various theories.

According to some hypotheses on IBS and functional dyspepsia (heartburn), the underlying cause of the disorder is the gut's defense mechanism against unconscious mental stress it does not want to cope with, or even directly confront, including negative emotions such as anger and anxiety. Rather than confront the stress and its underlying causes, the unconscious gut causes mild spasms in muscles and nerves, thereby causing symptoms. The conscious mind will therefore be distracted by these symptoms, enhancing the automatic repression process to keep the negative emotions contained in the unconscious body. (Remember, your body is your unconscious mind). This strategy keeps such emotional stress from surfacing in the conscious mind, thus assisting in the repression of painful emotions or anxiety and preventing awareness of them. The unconscious resembles a maximum security prison in this scenario.

CHAPTER 11

Stress, Skin Deep

The blush is beautiful, but it is sometimes convenient.
–Carlo Goldoni

The interaction between the mind and the skin is powerful. In fact, the mind may exert a greater influence on the skin than any other organ. Every day tens of thousands of dead skin cells shed as tiny flakes to allow cells at the bottom of the skin's epidermis to grow, move to the surface and differentiate into new skin cells. The constant renewal maintains the skin's permeability barrier to prevent the body's dehydration and protect against environmental irritants, infectious microbes. Like your body's other organs in the psychosomatic network, the skin uses messenger molecules to communicate with the brain and immune system. Research shows that psychological stress decreases cell growth and inhibits differentiation into skin cells. Blocking the stress hormone glucocorticoid prevents the inhibition.[195]

The skin is the largest organ (about 20 feet long if laid flat) and a very public venue where you willingly and unwillingly express emotion. An emerging medical specialty, "psychodermatologists" believe that psychological stress can exacerbate skin disorders, including hives, eczema, psoriasis, angioneurotic edema, urticaria (itching), acne, warts, rosacea and tattoos.

Yes, tattooing. Tattoos and piercing are popular art forms shared by people of all ages. Recent studies correlate no psychopathology in the self-expression of tattooing. In certain scenarios, however, tattoos can be indicative of a mind-body psychology of self-mutilation, defiance and independence from healthy societal norms. Prison and gang cultures use tattoos to signify their separation from "inferior" races, cultures or nationalities. Excessive adolescent tattooing can cross-over into pathological "cutting" which releases natural opiates that relieve tension but spur the addicting urge to do it again and again.

Tens of millions of Americans suffer from chronic skin ailments. Although many of these conditions have a physical trigger, the actual cause may be psychological. The patient's mind may create a nocebo expectation for painful symptoms to occur when a particular situation occurs. For example, some people expect to get a rash after exposure to cat hair. The irritant itself doesn't cause the skin to become irritated. Instead, the expectation of a reaction causes the breakout. Many psychogenic skin reactions start with either a personal or an environmental trigger. Traditional dermatologists customarily ignore the root cause of skin ailments and treat the obvious symptoms. Personal triggers could be anything from the stress of giving a speech or finishing a project with a deadline. Environmental triggers could be a bad smell, cat or dog hair, suspicious-looking substance or something else that makes people believe they have been exposed to an allergen, germ or a poison.

When an environmental trigger makes someone believe they might have been exposed to something dangerous, they may break out in hives. Hives are itchy, red skin rashes caused by histamines. Stress causes the release of histamines into the bloodstream, which can cause hives when they reach the skin. Some doctors even believe that repressing negative emotions like guilt or hostility can cause itching. A headache, dizziness, weakness or even a choking feeling may accompany skin reactions during emotional stress. Sometimes this is cause for immediate medical attention, as in the case of anaphylactic shock, a severe and potentially fatal allergic reaction that causes a dangerous drop in blood pressure, swelling and difficulty breathing. Call 911.

The skin is an organ connected to the physiology of the body as well as the mind. Under stress, the brain directs blood flow and nutrients to vital areas of the body. "Non-essential" organs, such as the skin receive less blood flow and nutrients, including oxygen. Chronic stress can lead to premature aging, making skin less supple, less hydrated and more prone to clogged pores and breakouts.

Psychogenic skin reactions are common, and can affect anyone under stress. Stress can even impair wound healing in some individuals. People channel psychological stress in different ways. Psychogenic skin reactions are not triggered by allergens or germs: the symptoms are caused by strong emotional reactions such as anxiety, excitement or anger, or by the fear of exposure to something harmful. Tension can delay the rate of waste removal from tissues and slow down skin cell turnover so the fresh epidermal cells take longer to reach the skin surface. Stress hormones such as cortisol also make the skin more vulnerable to environmental pollutants and germs. Chronic skin conditions are often resistant to conventional treatments. They require both conventional and complementary treatments. Antihistamines, behavioral therapy or assertiveness training are sometimes helpful.

Ted Grossbart, M.D., an assistant clinical professor of psychology at Harvard Medical School, has used visualization techniques with patients to help clear up plantar warts.[196] A few medical school dermatology programs have begun to provide skin stress-relief treatments. St. Luke's-Roosevelt Hospital in New York has a Psychocutaneous Medicine Unit where dermatologists and psychologists treat patients in tandem. The Johns Hopkins School of Medicine has a psychodermatology clinic where doctors recommend hypnosis or stress-reduction techniques for chronic skin ailments.[197] Meditation, breathing and other relaxation techniques can help tame the emotional reaction of the skin. Ayurvedic skin treatments have a definition of beauty that goes much deeper than the skin: a well-balanced diet, adequate sleep, stress management, exercise, and massage. While I would never recommend a trip to the tanning booth, investing time outdoors is a simple and inexpensive way to improve your appearance: ultraviolet light increases skin serotonin, a neurotransmitter that improves mood and resistance to stress.

The skin is the largest organ and one of the most sensitive to the effects of stress hormones. People have suspected a connection between skin disorders such as acne and stress. Research is finally proving a relationship. A recent study shows that emotional stress causes the hypothalamus, the brain's stress center, to release a chemical called corticotrophin-releasing hormone (CRH). Oil glands in the skin produce both CRH and CRH-receptors. When the CRH-receptors sense CRH, oil glands produce more oil, causing acne breakouts.[198]

The Science of Emotions and Health

Within the seemingly static tissue of the human body, cells work and communicate in a microscopic world that is constantly moving and changing. Factories inside our cells are directed by genes within the cell's nucleus which in turn are modulated by the molecules of emotion and cognition. With this knowledge, researchers are discovering the possible genetic and biochemical mechanisms underlying skin disease. Many of the nerve pathways and molecules underlying psychological responses and inflammatory disease are the same, making predisposition to one illness likely to go along with predisposition to another. The implications are profoundly important for preventing, managing and curing disease and illness. Psychogenic symptoms are not "all-in-your-head" or a sign of mental illness; they are the physiological manifestations of bodily systems that are not functioning well, and can function better with the therapies described in the next section of this book.

PART IV
Lasting Prescriptions

CHAPTER 12

Eastern Healing Traditions

Tension is who you think you should be. Relaxation is who you are.
– Chinese Proverb

Until the last century or so, doctors (and their predecessors, philosophers, priests and shamans, barbers and midwives) had little in their "black bags" except their compassion and humanity to heal. The healing touch, words of wisdom and spiritual practices such as prayer and meditation were woven together with the hope of creating lasting wellness. Now that prescriptions, tests and procedures have replaced the doctor-patient narrative, how can health care be more fulfilling? In Part III, we offer the best of holistic mind-body medicine mainly written by local experts in the field. Holistic medicine focuses on communication, compassion and treating "the whole person," instead of the disease or symptoms alone. Mind-body medicine can improve blood flow to the brain, help the body detoxify, put you on a better cycle of physical behavior, and decrease emotional stress. They also can improve thinking and mental function and decrease your tendency toward addiction. In short, mind-body practices are a lasting prescription.

Holistic medicine provides evidence-based and best practices for patient care. Evidence-based medicine means the conscientious, explicit, and judicious use of proven research in making decision about the care of individual patients. Previously accepted diagnostic tests and treatments will be replaced with new ones that are more powerful, more accurate, more efficacious, and safer. This is the role of holistic mind-body medicine today—it is becoming the medicine of tomorrow. Our journey begins where it all began—the ancient Far East.

Traditional Chinese Medicine

Heat from the Beijing sun began to clear the dust blowing in from the Gobi desert, but the congested streets of the ancient neighborhood remained a fog of purple haze, polluted from coal used to heat the buildings. Inside a medicinal garden beside a narrow alleyway, a woman with white hair met our Chinese guide, me and my daughter. She was caring for her feathered pets—several caged canaries hanging from the courtyard's trees and singing high-pitched songs.

My daughter's face was flushed a deep red: she was feverish and nauseous from malaria. When the woman saw her, she got down from her step-ladder and beckoned us to her "pharmacy," a single-story building with a green door and sign that read (in red Chinese characters), *Traditional Chinese Herbs*. Inside, the store's concrete floor was covered with dozens of air-tight containers and baskets of herbs. Two employees in tall white hats worked in the front room, mixing the herbs and preparing them in marked plastic bags on a long table with several trays. They stood in front of an impressive library of marked drawers. One of the pharmacists walked into the "boiler room" behind the counter where I could see "cooks" brewing herbs in pots on several burners. The strong smell forced me to sneeze and reminded me of the detestable kale my mother forced me to eat as a child.

Our guide explained that malaria has been treated for centuries in China with a common tea made from artemisinin, the active ingredient of the *qinghao* plant and named for "Artemisia," the Greek Goddess of Light. Bushy and barely three-feet high, the tree had tiny yellow flowers. The medicinal properties were concentrated in the leaves, which are shaped like ducks' feet.

Despite taking preventative anti-malarial drugs, my daughter had contracted the illness on our trip and was given the choice of conventional anti-malarial medicine or an herbal tea remedy with a 97 percent therapeutic success rate. Many herbs have been documented and well studied, although the World Health Organization (WHO) wouldn't approve artemisinin as a malaria treatment until 2001. She chose the tea as a preliminary cure and asked for a guide to the local herbal pharmacy.

It was October of 1999, and we were in Asia to celebrate the launch of AOL's Chinese edition, AOL Hong Kong through a partnership with China Internet Corp. (CIC), an affiliate of NASDAQ-traded China.com. AOL chief executive Steve Case joined the launch party at the Grand Hyatt Hong Kong overlooking the bedazzling Victoria Harbour. It was a defining moment like many other during the Internet age—the pinnacle of the world's largest communication medium, end of the millennium and dawn of the Chinese century where many new fortunes would be born.

I watched as the pharmacist took the *qinghao* or sweet wormwood leaves from a bulging burlap sack and weighed them on a brass hand-held scale. He then turned and entered the boiler room to prepare the tea, which had to be drunk several times a day, and within 24 hours of preparation. Although still nauseous, my daughter told me that she had recovered a certain clearness of mind after sipping the camphor-smelling tea.

As we discussed in the previous chapter on placebo, not everything can be explained naturally; many mysteries still exist in modern medicine, including the placebo effect of lesser herbs and supplements. And while you can't deny the healing power of herbs and supplements, you can't always trust their safety or effectiveness either.

With established anti-malarial medicines losing their effectiveness, the WHO recommended in 2001 that countries afflicted with malaria switch to a combination therapy based in part on the Chinese drug. Artemisinin-based drugs are the first Chinese pharmaceutical product to be broadly distributed internationally, beyond the more traditional remedies like ginseng.

According to the WHO, malaria is one of the most deadly diseases on the planet, with over 300 to 500 million persons infected every year. Although over 70 percent of deaths occur in Africa, almost half of the world's population that live in tropical or sub-tropical regions, including China, is at risk. Malaria is caused by plasmodium, a parasite that enters the human body through a mosquito bite. Inside the human host the parasite evades the immune system and quickly begins infecting the liver and red blood cells. Symptoms will appear about a week or two after the infectious mosquito bite: fever, headaches, vomiting, and a hot-cold torture of sweating and chills. If drugs are not available, the condition can become life-threatening. Malaria can kill by infecting and destroying red blood cells (leading to anemia) and by clogging the capillaries that carry blood to the brain (cerebral malaria) or other vital organs. The WHO estimates that malaria kills 2,000 African children each day.[199]

Over thirty years ago, Chairman Mao, who distrusted Western medicine, demanded that his scientists research Chinese history for home remedies. Scientists tested more than 200 herbs that had historically been used against malaria fevers. During that search they rediscovered the *Chinese Handbook of Prescriptions for Emergency Treatments* (340 AD) and found a 2,000-year-old recipe for a tea that claimed to cure malaria. The scientists refined the tea and extracted the active ingredient—artemisinin. Surprisingly, artemisinin has proven to be the most effective anti-malarial drug ever produced. But because of bitter Cold War rivalries and secrecy, the remedy's introduction to the global community took several decades.

In recent years, the popular media that connects our global community through the Internet, television and more artistic mediums such as literature and film have advanced our understanding and appreciation of Eastern culture. Our radically different ways of looking at life and mind have existed apart over a span of almost 2,500 years. Today, the development of technical inventions have drawn us closer to each other, so East and West are no longer separated by almost insurmountable voids of time and distance.

Eastern philosophers have been thinking about consciousness for centuries. The mystical tradition behind traditional Chinese medicine (TCM) teaches that the mind and body belong to an indivisible continuum. Traditions such as Judaism, Christianity and Islam separate the realms of the body and the soul. In the metaphysical context, the "soul," "spirit" and "mind" are interchangeable terms. If you think in Western dualistic terms, the mind or soul is the thing that does the thinking and feeling and can exist apart from the brain. Psychological states and changes in neurobiological properties that we can observe and quantify are beginning to bridge this divide. Eastern mystics claim to discover God in the depths of their being while the Christian looks to the righteousness of Christ Jesus.

Harmony Within

Traditional Chinese Medicine (TCM) based on the teachings of Buddhism, Taoism and Confucianism rejects any dualism of mind and body and considers the body as the temple, energy as the force, and spirit as the governor of life. When the spirit takes command, the body naturally follows it. This arrangement benefits all three. However, when the body leads the way, the spirit goes along, and this harms all three.[200]

In TCM, health is taught as "harmony within the body as well as between the body and the universe." To be healthy, the body needs to be in balance, as does the world around it. Thoughts and feelings are considered vital to maintaining bodily health. Behaviors and relationships directly impact health.

People who practice TCM believe that the body's vital energy (*chi*) circulates through channels called "meridians" that have branches connected to bodily organs and functions. Illness is attributed to imbalance or interruption of *chi*. When a TCM doctor prescribes a specific herb, she's not attempting to correct a chemical dysfunction; rather, she's trying to restore the harmonious flow of chi.

The first Yellow Emperor, Huang Di, was the author of the classic *Traditional Chinese Medicine* (2500 BC). TMC is an integral part of Chinese culture. Diet and herbs, massage and manipulation, and martial arts like Tai Chi and Qigong are still popular today. Chinese physicians also use acupuncture, a medical procedure involving insertion and manipulation of needles to treat pain or various conditions.

Tao, the Way

Taoism, the popular Chinese way of life associated with TCM, teaches that disease evolves from cosmic imbalances of the yin and the yang, opposite poles of nature that are complimentary, not conflicting. The yang transforms and the yin conserves. Emotions are the balance of yin and yang in humans and have the potential to produce profound physiological effects. According to Taoism, all change is cyclical and predictable. Everything from a woman's menstrual cycle, the sexual behavior of men and animals or the cosmic forces of night and day, life and death are predictable. Without polarity the world and universe as we know it could not exist. The terms "yin" and "yang" first appeared in the *Chinese Book of Change* circa 1250 AD.[201]

> The ceaseless interplay of heaven and earth gives form to all things. The sexual union of male and female gives life to all things. The interaction of yin and yang is called the Way (Tao), and the resulting creative process is called change.[202]

The influence of Taoism on Chinese civilization has been second only to that of Confucianism. The definition of Taoism is the philosophy of simplicity and non-interference. In the Taoist view, healing must begin with the individual's conscious refusal to participate in the stressful and aggressive ways of life. Healthy individuals seek to fulfill their potential harmony with the Tao by a quiet and sensitive contemplation of the natural tendency in things—

the yin and the yang—making their life like a smooth-flowing river, clear and undisturbed. Taoist believers are to relate to other people in a spirit of natural kindness, tolerance, and humility, never striving to dominate them.

Acupuncture

Acupuncture is a conservative form of treatment for acute or chronic pain, and is performed by trained medical providers who typically spend more time with the patient than traditional physicians. Acupuncturists perform a thorough physical exam, taking pulses, feeling the texture of the skin and taking a complete psychological history. Although an acupuncturist isn't a medical doctor, the National Commission for the Certification of Acupuncture developed an exam to certify qualified candidates in the field. In recent years, the popularity of acupuncture has doubled in the US. Today, Americans can seek an acupuncturist in most communities.

Acupuncture shares the same basic tenets of TCM, including chi, yin and yang, internal and external cause of disease, lifestyle, and meridians. The goal of acupuncture is to promote the flow of chi—life energy—through the body by redirecting energy that's "stuck." The acupuncture points are like gates with locks; inserting the acupuncture instrument at the correct point opens or frees the energy to balance the vital polarity of the yin and the yang. Acupuncture has been scientifically proven to treat a host of common disorders, including chronic back pain, skin disorders and carpal tunnel syndrome.

The ancient Daoists of China, along with the influence of health traditions from other Asian countries, developed several ways to assist in achieving and maintaining health. They used diet and herbs, Qigong (meditation, breathing, and exercises), bodywork (massage and acupressure), and acupuncture. They also stressed the study of Feng Shui and the Classics, such as the I Ching and Dao de Ching.

Acupressure is based on the same theories as acupuncture; however, in acupressure, acu-points are held with fingers and thumbs rather than putting needles in. While acupuncture is highly effective for many health issues, acupressure is more effective for stress and tension related problems. Both work by balancing the energy and by releasing endorphins. However, acupressure also helps to release muscular tension as many of the points are on muscles, thus the client receives many of the benefits of both massage and acupuncture. Another advantage of acupressure is that anyone can learn simple points they can use at home for self-acupressure. Some forms of acupressure such as Jin Shin Do are especially helpful for facilitating emotional release, as emotions are held in the body and can be a factor in many health issues.

Qigong

Qigong is a gentle yet effective program for improving our health and energy through simple stretches and exercises, breathing and relaxation, self-acupressure and massage, visualization, and meditation. The gentle, rhythmic movements of Qigong reduce stress, build stamina, increase vitality, and enhance the immune system. Many who practice Qigong regularly find that it helps them regain a youthful vitality, maintain health even into old age and speed recovery from illness.

Qigong is grounded in the ancient Chinese Daoist philosophy and is confirmed by Western scientific research to have a number of health benefits, including reducing hypertension and the incidence of falling in the aged population. It has also been found to improve cardiovascular, respiratory, circulatory, lymphatic and digestive functions. People do Qigong to maintain health, heal their bodies, calm their minds, and reconnect with their spirit. Qigong's great appeal is that anyone can benefit, from the most physically challenged to the super athlete, regardless of ability, age, belief system or life circumstances. Since Qigong can be practiced anywhere or at any time, there is no need to buy special clothing or equipment or to join a health club.

The name "Qigong" is derived from two Chinese characters. The first is Qi, meaning life force or energy. The second character, "gong," means practice or cultivation. "Gong" is sometimes translated as "work," but I prefer "practice" since I don't see it as work but as fun! Taiji (often spelled T'ai Chi), which is a form of Qigong, is translated as the Supreme Ultimate. Quan (or Chuan) means boxing or fist. Using the term Taiji is commonly used today to refer to the health practice while using the term Taiji Quan is most often used in reference to the martial art form.

Taiji is considered the "supreme ultimate" because it goes right to the root of most health problems by relaxing the body and the mind, aligning the spine, promoting deep breathing and balancing the energy systems. In modern terms, Tai Chi and Qigong could be considered ancient systems of biofeedback and classical conditioning.

Qigong is divided into 2 main categories: active/dynamic and tranquil/passive. In general, you could say that "active" is exercise and "passive" is meditation, though there is not a strict boundary between the two. Exercise, or active, can be further divided into health practices and martial arts, with Taiji being both. Meditation, or passive, can be further divided into active meditation, such as visualization, and passive or tranquil meditation, which is emptying the mind. The most important goal of meditation is to achieve a tranquil, calm mind, which was believed to be necessary for spiritual enlightenment. You can do Qigong meditation sitting, standing, and laying down, walking or during moving exercises such as Taiji. Further, once you have developed the Qi in your own body-mind, you can then utilize this energy for external healing on others, or internally, to heal your own body.

CHAPTER 13

Mindful Meditation

It is not the brains that matter most, but that which guides them—
the character, the heart, generous qualities, progressive ideas.
– Fyodor Dostoyevsky

Meditation has a pervasive effect on stress. The practice promotes a fundamental detachment from the future, the past, and the material world by freeing the mind of imagination and all thoughts. Most forms of meditation seek to quiet the internal chatter that prevents us from entering into a state of deep relaxation. Herbert Benson, MD ran experiments on volunteers who sat quietly for 20 minutes while he and his colleagues hooked them up to heart, brain and breathing monitors. After fitting them with the measurement devices, he asked them to meditate for 20 minutes and then shift their focus to every day thoughts for another 20 minutes. The results were dramatic—all involuntary physiological activity in the brain, heart and lungs slowed down during the meditative session but remained the same during the pre and post-meditative periods.[202]

From a physiological perspective, meditation induces a deep state of relaxation, including a lower metabolism, heart rate, breathing rate and the activation of various brain regions associated with positive emotional states. Meditation quiets the frontal cortex, the executive center of the brain that regulates our daily thoughts, emotions, plans and actions. Quieting this area of the brain triggers a soothing release of chemicals from the brain's emotional centers. Meditation creates a hypnotic state deeper than sleep that also drops blood lactate, a maker of stress and anxiety. People who practice meditation daily can lower their risk of hypertension and heart disease and reduce dependency on pain medication.

Meditation has both physiological and psychological benefits. People who meditate can become more aware of the distorted aspects of their individual view of human experience. Mark Epstein, MD, psychiatrist and meditation practitioner compares it to looking directly at a star at night. It's difficult to see the shape clearly until you look away slightly. He believes meditation can be used to calm narcissistic tendencies. In Greek mythology, Narcissus stood for vanity, callousness and insensitivity. Focusing on the word, "love" or "compassion" can train the mind to see others in a more positive light.

Developing a here and now, moment-to-moment capacity of mind allows the self to be experienced without idealization—without narcissistic distortions. For example, we often feel as if we must *express* our emotions, because simply knowing the feeling is an idea that doesn't usually occur to us. Meditative techniques teach us to "be" with the full range of our human emotions instead of rushing to express, numb or exorcise them. The practice doesn't require people to deny their emotions, only to learn to experience them in a new way. Psychotherapy can help identify negative subconscious emotions, attitudes, and beliefs and help control erotic and aggressive behavior, but it has not been able to deliver freedom from narcissistic cravings in the search for lasting satisfaction.[204] Meditation offers a lasting, sustaining peace.

Our culture teaches us that we must control or suppress our feelings rather than acknowledge them. Rather than accepting ourselves, we often want to fix or change things. Meditation is "critical mental development" (not intellectual development, such as studying facts or ideas). It teaches us how to empty our mind of thoughts so we can create "thoughts without a thinker." By focusing the mind on just one thing, people who practice meditation can attain a deeper level of insight about themselves and the human condition. "When the mind exists undisturbed in the way, nothing in the world can offend, and when a thing can no longer offend, it ceases to exist."[205] Meditation has a calming effect that allows you to transcend the day-to-day, month-to-month or lifetime disappointments. It can be a form of loving God, achieving mental peace or psychological insight, and can reduce stress and even enhance athletic or artistic performance.

One Breath at a Time

To begin meditating, sit in a comfortable position in a quiet place and close your eyes. As relaxation ability improves, meditation can occur within a shorter period of time, but try a half hour initially. Breathing is critical in meditation. Concentrating on the in and out of breathing is a sharp contrast to the cluttered thinking of our daily minds. Deep breathing releases calming endorphins. Take two to three deep breaths in through your nose for an immediate release of tension. For deeper relaxation, take seven to eight breaths from your belly. This is deep, abdominal breathing, and lightheadedness can occur if you get up too quickly.

To calm your mind, you may choose to focus on your feet, slowing moving up to each body part, ending at the top of your head. Choose a focus word or phrase that reflects your belief system and silently repeat it on each exhalation. For example, Christians may repeat the prayer, "Lord Jesus Christ, have mercy on me." Jews may repeat "shalom" or "create a new heart in me." You may also choose to focus on repetition of a word such as "compassion" or "love." Other people may want to concentrate on a picture or on a spot on the wall. The most popular Eastern mantra is "Ong, Namo Guru Dee Namo." Vibrations from repeated mantras can affect activity in the endocrine system, including the brain's pituitary and hypothalamus.

Meditation is taking consciousness and all its thoughts and creating a state of tranquility. It is counter-culture. If your mind wanders during your meditation, redirect your concentration to your breathing. Don't judge or worry about the fact that your mind drifted. Tell yourself, "Okay" or "Oh, well" and continue with the meditation. Avoid peripheral thinking such as "I need to take out the garbage" or "my project is due next Thursday," and so on.

Within the core of many of the world's spiritual traditions are forms of meditation that allow the practitioner to access a deeper level of spiritual consciousness. God commands His people to meditate on His word day and night to instill obedience. The Judeo-Christian Bible uses the words *mediate* or *meditation* twenty times. Meditation can center Christians, Muslims, Hindi and Jews by focusing attention on a repeated prayer, mantra, sound or object such as the rosary. Many kinds of meditation exist, including Zen, Buddhist, Transcendental, Christian, and more.

"Mindful" meditation is a technique to gain psychological wisdom and insight. Instead of ignoring distracting thoughts, you focus on them. According to Jon Kabat-Zinn, this form of meditation practice can cultivate a greater awareness of the human experience, helping people live each moment as fully as possible. It can teach people to deal more effectively with stress or painful life situations by confronting negative emotions and accepting them rather than avoiding or repressing them. Personal growth comes from observing, not judging or analyzing your thoughts as they occur during the meditation. This can help you feel less caught up in any negative thoughts, fears or pressures such as chronic illness. It allows you to step back and see more clearly what's on your mind or what drives you.

An excellent CD-Rom that teaches meditation is Andrew Weil and Jon Kabat-Zinn's *Meditation for Optimum Health*. To practice mindful meditation, follow the same steps as noted earlier in the chapter but when you begin to lose focus and think about an approaching deadline, memory, or feeling in your body or mind, note it before returning to your primary meditative focus. Observing your thoughts, feelings and sensations can lead to personal insights that provide a more lucid picture of your mind and its activities. This "way of being" teaches you to become more aware and in touch with your mind and body in the present moment. You may begin to feel more confident about your response to stressful situations. Pain may become less threatening, and more of an opportunity for personal growth. The regular practice of mindful meditation can reduce the degree of suffering inherent to the human condition.

Taoist Buddhism

Religious Taoism has merged with Buddhism and other religions in China. Buddhism, a major world religion, began in northeastern India with the teachings of Siddhartha Gautama, known as the Buddha, or Enlightened One. At the core of the Buddha's enlightenment was his realization of the *Four Noble Truths*:

1) Life is suffering. Human existence is painful from the moment of birth to the moment of death. Even death brings no relief, for the Buddha believed the Hindu idea of life as cyclical, with death leading to further rebirth.

2) All suffering is caused by ignorance of the nature of reality, and the craving, attachment, and grasping that result from such ignorance.

3) Suffering can be ended by overcoming ignorance and attachment to material things.

4) The path to the suppression of suffering is the Noble Eightfold Path: right views, right intention, right speech, right action, right livelihood, right effort, right-minded-ness, and right contemplation. These eight concepts are

divided into three categories that form the cornerstone of Buddhist faith: morality, wisdom, and concentration.[206]

Zen is a form of Chinese Buddhism that emphasizes meditation and insight as a way to enlightenment or spiritual awakening. Zen Buddhism originated in twelfth-century China and emphasizes meticulous daily practice and retreats. Practicing with others is valued as a way to avoid the traps of ego. Vulnerability cultivates humility. Zen teachers have frequently made the point that meditation isn't a state of consciousness, it is a *way of life*: a life of humility; a life of labor; a life of service; a life of prayer and gratitude; and a life of meditation. "A day without work is a day without eating," according to one of the tenets of Zen.

According to Buddha, "All worry about the self is vain; the ego is like a mirage, and all the tribulations that touch it will pass away." Buddha teaches that individuals who "awaken" through meditation are free of fear. In Buddhism, meditation is an attempt to break through and expose narcissism. Freud recognized that the inability to tolerate unpleasant truths about oneself was essential to narcissism. Two of the humiliations we try to avoid as humans are illness and death. Zen meditation can be used to free the mind of addiction, compulsive and obsessive behaviors, and fear of pain, illness and death by leading to a life of moderation. Zen Buddhism is less about religion and more about a practical methodology for psychological relief.

The mind is the constantly changing flow of molecular information in motion throughout the body. Exhalation during meditation quiets the activity of many nerve cells. Expiration slows the firing of nerve cells in the amygdala. Meditation to enlightenment begins with acknowledging that you need nothing from the outside. Food and drink do not bring ultimate satisfaction. Controlling your mind can lead to better behavior, according to Zen teachings. Freud's theories dovetail with Buddhism, in that the pursuit of pleasurable sensory experiences is unsustainable. "What is the Noble Truth of the Extinction of Suffering?" asked the Buddha. "It is the complete fading away and extinction of craving, its forsaking and abandonment, liberation and detachment from it."[206]

Popular, powerful antidepressants or sedatives don't have to be the first and only answer doctors provide for anxiety or depression. In fact, the conclusion of recent brain scans on people who meditate is that through training the mind, people can become calmer, especially those who suffer from emotional ups and downs.[207] People who struggle with stress-related disease or destructive emotions can reprogram their brain through meditative techniques that foster more enduring transformations of personality than short-term pharmaceutical effects.

Tibetan Buddhists

Tibetan Buddhists believe the Dalai Lama to be one of innumerable incarnations of Avalokitesvara who embodies the compassion of all Buddhas. According to classic Buddhist texts, the benefits of meditating on compassion include loving and being loved by people and animals, having a serene mind, sleeping and waking peacefully, and enjoying pleasant dreams.

If you have a sense of caring for others, you will manifest a kind of inner strength in spite of your own difficult situations and problems. With this strength, your problems will seem less significant and bothersome. By going beyond your own problems and taking care of others, you gain inner strength, self-confidence, courage, and a greater sense of calm. This is a clear example of how one's way of thinking can really make a difference.[209]

The daily act of meditating on others' well-being is similar to the Judeo-Christian practice of prayer that can create a state of emotional, mental and spiritual calmness and joy.

As we learned in the chapter on biochemistry, the brain regulates thought and emotions, but isn't the single sight of the psyche. Emotions are present throughout the body's blood, organs, muscles, bones and skin. The mind doesn't dominate the body—it becomes the body; the body and the mind are one. The molecules of emotion are stored in the body and can either circulate or be stored away in the subconscious. Meditation can reprogram your biochemistry and strengthen your mind-body and mental apparatus. It can cultivate an inner wakefulness with no object of thought or perception, just pure consciousness aware of its own unbounded nature. It is wholeness, aware of itself, devoid of differences, suffering or criticism. The practice of meditation increases patience, compassion, and other virtues and morals that promote peace or bring people closer together and closer to God.

CHAPTER 14

Ayurvedic Medicine

As is a man's will, so is his action. As is his action, so he becomes.
–Brihadaranyaka Upanisad

The most renowned Indian system of preventative medicine and health care is Ayurveda, "the science of a long life." Ayurveda advocates a specific holistic lifestyle, along with therapeutic practices that promote physical, mental, social and spiritual harmony. Today Ayurvedic hospitals and practitioners are flourishing throughout India. In the United States, Ayurveda is popular at luxury spas and health resorts where the treatments promote relaxation of mind and body, as well as physical rejuvenation. Dating back more than 5,000 years, ancient Ayurvedic texts teach that three energies create all life: "vata," "pitta," and "kapha."

Vata is the energy responsible for movement and creativity. Pitta is responsible for transformations, such as courage, digestion and metabolism. Kapha rules structures and affects things like growth, fluids, and compassion. According to the Ayurvedic philosophy, everyone has a predominant mind-body type, or "dosha" of vata, pitta or kapha that influences everything from health to appearance and personality.[210] Ancient Ayurveda claims that disease and illness result from an imbalance of the doshas, but has also adopted many Western ideas related to the root of illness such as pathogens, infectious agents and genetic predisposition.

Ayurvedic physicians try to view sickness in the context of the patient's life, drawing upon a broad range of approaches to awaken and support a person's inner healing response. Unlike Western medicine, Ayurvedic treatments focus on disease prevention, including recommendations for diet, stress management, exercise, emotional healing, nutritional and herbal supplements, and sensory modulation. Ayurvedic practitioners also recognize the constitutional differences between individuals, as well as the changes that occur in people at different times in their lives. If indicated, practitioners can also recommend more aggressive tactics for management of disease.

Ayurveda, as a holistic system, recommends a lifestyle that is conducive to mental peace and clarity. To achieve optimum wellness, according to Ayurvedic texts, harmony must exist between mental and physical actions, mind and body.[211] On a philosophical level, Ayurveda urges one to embrace universal human values such as non-violence, chastity, honesty, compassion, and equanimity. Beauty, according to Ayurvedic philosophy, reflects compassion and energy flowing more freely through the body that in turn results in less tension in the face, and a reduction in wrinkle lines.

The meditation, yoga and breathing exercises advocated in Ayurveda are thought to lead to better mental health through stress reduction. "Ultimately the best use of a physician's knowledge is to teach people how to heal themselves," according to Ayurvedic physician David Simon, M.D. Ayurvedic practices can reduce the worsening physical effects of diseases such as hypertension, diabetes, cardiovascular disease, Crohn's disease and other conditions exacerbated by stress.

Like Traditional Chinese Medicine, Ayurvedic physicians focus on rituals involving astrology or cosmic balance and apply hundreds of herbal medicines. Ayurveda also teaches that 107 "marmas" exist in the body, (similar to the meridian points of Chinese medicine). Oil-based massage and herbs can release toxins and help restore the normal energy flow of the marmas. Ayurvedic treatments don't carry the toxic side-effects of many Western prescriptions. The subtle benefits take a long time to accumulate.

Ayurveda promotes a diet rich in organic and natural foods, mild herbs, regular exercise and mental health measures such as yoga. In addition to dietary recommendations, Ayurveda prescribes guidelines for proper food consumption, including the appropriate quantity, frequency and timing of food intake. Ayurveda also teaches basic lifestyle habits such as proper rest, regular massage and external application of essential oils to enhance elasticity of the muscles and ligaments. Some of the advantages of massage are pain relief, improved circulation, stress relief, better sleep, flexibility, and emotional release. People can also enjoy the cosmetic benefits of massage, warm stones and oils that create a refreshing glow to the skin.

Deepak Chopra is perhaps the best-known Ayurvedic teacher and practitioner. In his best-selling book, *Perfect Health*, Chopra tells us how our lives can be influenced, extended and ultimately controlled without interference from illness and old age. A guiding principle of Ayurveda is that the mind asserts the greatest influence on the body; freedom from sickness depends on your own conscious awareness and emotional and spiritual balance. "The Ayurvedic sages teach that there is an impulse in all of us to grow and progress. This impulse governs our overall balance automatically; it can be seen at work in every cell, but particularly in the brain …"[212] Ayurvedic medicine address a person's health concerns from a physical, emotional and spiritual perspective. Integrating the theoretical frameworks of Ayurveda and modern science, the physicians focus as much on the person who is facing a health challenge as the health challenge being faced.

Anatomy of Back Pain

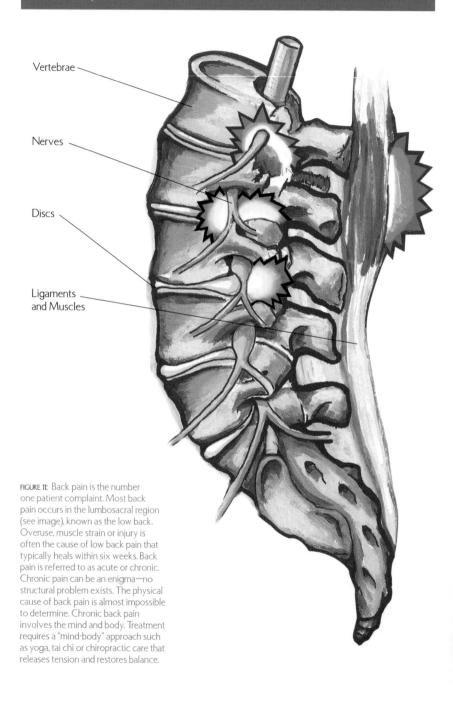

Vertebrae

Nerves

Discs

Ligaments
and Muscles

FIGURE 11: Back pain is the number
one patient complaint. Most back
pain occurs in the lumbosacral region
(see image), known as the low back.
Overuse, muscle strain or injury is
often the cause of low back pain that
typically heals within six weeks. Back
pain is referred to as acute or chronic.
Chronic pain can be an enigma—no
structural problem exists. The physical
cause of back pain is almost impossible
to determine. Chronic back pain
involves the mind and body. Treatment
requires a "mind-body" approach such
as yoga, tai chi or chiropractic care that
releases tension and restores balance.

CHAPTER 15

The Healing Touch of Chiropractic Care
By James M. Cox

*Chiropractic is based on the premise that the body possesses an
internal system that strives for balance. This internal system is
called your innate intelligence.*
—Robert Berkowitz, D.C.

Chiropractic care seeks to restore balance to the nervous system
through manipulation of the spinal column and other body structures.
Daniel David Palmer developed chiropractic care in the late
nineteenth century based on a systematic study of anatomy,
physiology, and healing arts from around the world. Chiropractic is
the largest and most popular branch of complementary medicine that
offers simple, safe, proven procedures to relieve back pain.

A study in the *NEJM* reported that from 1990-1993, more people
visited holistic health providers than all primary care medical
providers nationwide. The trend continues today. Nearly half of
patients seek out complementary care, and both patients and
physicians voice increasing dissatisfaction with the practice of
mainstream medicine. Patients fear telling their medical doctor about
their decision to seek alternative care because they fear a negative
response. Patients don't feel angry at their medical doctor; they just
want help and cooperation between health care providers. Today
patients want, and demand more than a prescription for increasingly
more powerful drugs and more expensive diagnostic testing that fails
to relieve their pain; rather it increases their frustration.

Chiropractic emphasizes that there's no distinction between mind
and body. One key property of chiropractic practice is touch and
palpation in the examination and treatment of the patient. The word
chiropractic is derived from the Greek words "chiro" and "prakticos,"
meaning "hand practitioner." Chiropractors touch people and people,
especially those in pain, find it pain relieving and relaxing. The very
theory of chiropractic practice is to relieve nerve interference in the

spine that can be caused by pinched nerves, arthritis, disc herniation, spinal stenosis, or other mechanical problems. Chiropractic philosophy credits innate intelligence (the inherent ability of the body to heal itself) as a necessary basis for its clinical outcome success. Chiropractors manipulate the human spine to release nerve pressure on spinal nerves, relax muscles, and create normal nerve conduction from the extremities and spine to flow to the spinal cord and brain; anyone recognizes this benefit by the mere act of massage and its relaxing feeling. It is relaxing and soothing to the nervous system. Further explanation of the benefits of chiropractic manipulation includes that it produces a drop in pressure inside the intervertebral disc when the spine receives manipulation; there is increase in the size of the nerve openings in the spine, and reduced chemical inflammation around nerves in and exiting the spinal cord. Recent research has shown that spinal manipulation reduces pain caused by chemically inflamed spinal nerves.[213]

Comparison of Chiropractic with Other Forms of Treatment

A recent comparative study of chiropractic spinal manipulation to exercise for treating chronic low back pain found chiropractic manipulation to be the superior form of care, especially in treating patients with low back and lower extremity pain.[214] Another study showed that in a 1000 case study of low back and leg pain patients, 91 percent of patients attained maximum relief of their pain within 90 days of care and 43 percent required up to 10 chiropractic visits.[215] Another study showed that 76 percent of lumbar stenosis patients showed relief of pain and 73 percent showed improvement in disability following chiropractic spinal manipulation.[216] Sixty-eight patients with mild to moderate degenerative disc changes in the neck causing pain and weakness were randomized to two treatment groups: conservative care with manipulation, exercise, soft collar, medication or surgical care. No significant differences in deterioration or superior outcome between the two groups were reported.[217]

Chiropractors, in addition to spinal and body manipulation, instruct patients in exercise, nutrition, and the value of healthy living via instructional programs like Back School. Back School is a class to teach patients the anatomy of the spine, the generators of pain in the spine that cause pain, and ergonomics which is the lifting and bending laws of every day work to prevent back pain. The class stresses that there is often no cure for back pain, but back pain can be controlled through proper daily activities of living that do not cause stress to the spine.

Patient care with chiropractic encompasses, in addition to the physical benefits of touch and manipulation, the person's feelings, thoughts, and spiritual principles. In discussing history and examination findings with patients, personal facts about their emotional history often arise. For some, it may be the first time they discuss such past issues as child abuse, neglect, emotional abuse, marital unrest, children issues, unresolved family disagreements, past mistakes, sexual abuse, parental issues, religious spiritual unrest, etc. Without addressing the feelings created by these dysfunctional parts of their lives, patients cannot strive for the balance of memory, emotion, and thought that creates the feeling of wellbeing we term homeostasis, or put another way—the Mind, Body and Spirit connection. The chiropractor who listens, touches, and balances these three aspects of the human condition can often help patients as much or more than drugs and surgery.

Touch and personal time with the patient under chiropractic care is proven. More than 88 million visits for care of back and neck pain were made to chiropractors and 10 million to massage, relaxation techniques, and yoga in 1997. Two of three users preferred chiropractic or massage and one in four preferred conventional medical doctors.[218]

Why does the number of patients seeking chiropractic care continue to increase? Simple—they feel better. The chiropractor spends time in examining and explaining the patient's problem. He or she touches them—sometimes the only exposure some patients have to the sedation of human touch. If the chiropractor can talk in a friendly, helpful, caring voice, he or she will gain the patient's trust and confidence. Chiropractors listen not only for the content of the patient's narrative but for the expressive cues—images, associated subplots, silences, where he or she chooses to begin in telling of him or herself, how he or she sequences symptoms with other life events. Patients will raise a low spiritual energy level which is a feeling of fear, worry, anger, frustration, bitterness, resentment, and hopelessness to the higher spiritual energy level of peace, confidence, hope, joy, forgiveness, kindness, love, and happiness.[219] A Lutheran minister once said that if he were in one room counseling patients on their spiritual life, and a chiropractor was performing adjustments in the next room, they could treat most human illness. He was right. There is not question that a kind word, a touch, a soothing remark, and a chiropractic spinal adjustment to relieve stress and nerve tension is a positive step in a patient's life. They bear the burden of the patient's suffering.

Contrast of Chiropractic Care and Western Medical Care

Most medical doctors' care of spine pain does not involve touch. Traditional treatment is drugs, epidural steroid injections, facet joint steroid injections, and surgery; all of which involve little if any touch between the physician and the patient's painful body. The typical patient visits a chiropractor after seeing their general practitioner for back pain who prescribes drugs such as non-steroidal inflammatory drugs, pain killers, muscle relaxants, narcotic drugs, and finally may order an MRI of the spine to identify any obvious pain generating problems. The general practitioner then refers the patient to either a physical therapist for electrical stimulation, exercises, massage, heat, cold, etc. or else refers the patient to a neurosurgeon or orthopedic surgeon. Here the surgeon may recommend epidural steroid drugs, more therapy, trigger point or facet joint injections, stronger drugs, or surgery.

An example of questionable spine pain treatment is the epidural steroid injection. Epidural steroid injections into inflamed nerves are very popular today and are a non touch form of care. Studies show that 32 percent receiving them will report more than two months pain relief, 39 percent report less than 2 months of relief, and 29 percent report no pain relief.[220] The placebo effect of epidural steroid injections is suggested by the findings of a study showing that three epidural injections with salt water gave the same relief of sciatic pain as did steroid used in the injection.[221]

It is usually after the patient exhausts these medical therapies that chiropractors are consulted by the patient—as a last-ditch effort to avoid surgery. Now please note that surgery is sometimes the answer, but in only 1 – 2 percent of back pain patients is surgery necessary. That leaves the other 98 percent to be treated with the best non-surgically evidence based care such as chiropractic. The federal government in 1994 stated spinal manipulation should be the first clinical treatment for back pain and the American Academy of Orthopedic Surgeons list chiropractic care as an approach to treating spinal stenosis. Chiropractors perform 94 percent of the spinal manipulation done in the US.

Surgical Compared with Non-Surgical Care of Spine Pain

Medical studies show that surgical treatment of spine pain often is not better than non surgical care. For example, the Maine Lumbar Spine Study showed that the ten-year outcome of treating sciatica caused by herniated disc, which is the most common cause of leg pain in the adult working populations, that 69 percent of surgically treated and 61 percent of non-surgically treated sciatic disc herniated patients were improved. The same study of spinal stenosis induced leg pain patients showed about 50 percent of both the surgically and non surgically treated patients were improved.[222] Note that this also means 50 percent of stenosis patients were not improved by surgery and 30 to 40 percent of herniated disc cases were still in pain. The long term outcome of surgery and non-surgery care for back and leg pain is equal, but both far from giving total relief. Approximately half of these back and leg pain patients continue to have their pain. I say that we do not cure back pain and leg pain, *we control it* and this requires cooperation between the doctor and the patient, whether the doctor is a medical doctor or chiropractic doctor.

Today we see extensive spinal fusion surgeries with poorly shown positive outcomes. A study in the *British Medical Journal* in 2005 found that no clear outcome was seen between primary spinal fusion surgery and intensive rehabilitation in patients with chronic low back pain.[223] The cost of treating back pain is staggering: in 1998 it was reported that the cost for office visits for back pain was $11.1 billion; $4.5 billion for hospitalization; $3.9 billion for prescription drugs; $4.7 billion for outpatient services; and $1.1 billion for emergency room care. The total, $26 billion was up from $20 billion in 1984, a 30 percent increase.

Yet, studies show there is little evidence that patients are better off for all the treatment. Surgery is under new scrutiny with a national study of 1000 patients with disc herniation or spinal stenosis (narrowing of the spinal canal that usually results from arthritis, aging, and degenerative spondylolisthesis) who were randomly assigned to have surgery or not. The study, reported in *JAMA* found that people with ruptured discs in their lower backs usually recover whether or not they have surgery. Surgery appeared to relieve pain more quickly but most people recovered eventually and that there was no harm in waiting. James N. Weinstein, M.D., a professor of orthopedic surgery and community and family medicine at Dartmouth medical school and editor of *Spine* journal, one of the investigators of the study, said some surgeons fear the study may take away their practice of surgery.[224] All of the fusion surgeries being done today carry with them a high price tab in human suffering and dollars when they are not successful.

CHAPTER 16

Breath Is the Key to Emotional Control

Breath is the link between the body and mind, and between the conscious and unconscious mind. It is the master key to the control of emotions and to operations of the autonomic nervous system.
—Andrew Weil

The single most effective relaxation technique is the conscious regulation of breath. When we breathe, oxygen enters the blood stream in the lungs through the alveolar sacs, and attaches to the hemoglobin. When a cell receives oxygen, it also expels carbon dioxide through exhalation. The diaphragm contracts at the base of the lungs and air pressure fills the lungs. Many different types of breathing techniques exist, but I recommend four basic techniques: complete breath, alternate nasal breath, fire breathing (Lamaze), and one-minute breath.

An effective breathing technique employed by athletes in high performance workouts involves breathing through the nose while exercising to increase lung capacity. This technique is based on the Indian principle that oxygen is the transporter of "prana," or life force. Prana is said to travel to the brain along the olfactory nerve. Prana nourishes the control centers in the brain, and energizes the deepest levels of the lungs and blood stream, thereby enhancing workouts.

The breath is the secret to meditation. To begin, use a complete breath. Breathe deeply starting with the belly and diaphragm. Feel the air going through your nostrils, in and out. After about 10-20 deep breaths, your blood pressure and heart rate will decrease, electrical brain patterns will change, and your perception of pain will be less. You will also feel calm. Breathing affects your pain threshold via the periaqueductal gray or PAG, your pleasure and pain network which is densely packed with receptors for endorphins. By breathing deeply, rapidly or holding your breath, you can increase the natural endorphins in your lungs and brain. Breath is the master key to the control of emotions and operations of the autonomic nervous system.

Conventional therapies are available for most sleep disorders, but for some people they don't work well and cause unwanted side effects. Over 26 million Americans take a popular sleep-aide, despite side-effects linked to binge-eating, hallucinations and violent outbursts. Among sleep-eaters taking sleep aides, the desire for food can be tremendously powerful. The medication causes the brain to intertwine the basic instincts of sleeping with eating. According to *The New York Times*, one woman who started taking Ambien while recovering from back surgery began to notice that food was missing from her refrigerator:

> She accused two nursing aides who were caring for her of
> stealing food. It was not until her son came to spend several
> nights that she realized that despite the body cast, she was
> getting up to eat while she was asleep. The first night her
> son was there, he found her standing in the kitchen, body
> cast and all, frying bacon and eggs. The next night he found
> her eating a sandwich, and sent her back to bed. Later that
> same night, her son arose to find her standing in the kitchen
> again. "I had turned the oven on," she recalled. "I store pots
> and pans in the oven and I had turned it to 500 degrees."[225]

According to the NIH, up to 70 million Americans (almost one out of three adults) have some kind of sleep problem.[226] Breathing exercises can induce deep states of relaxation and release of tension after a stressful day. Slow, smooth breathing counteracts anxious thoughts that sometimes keep sleep at bay. And the exercises won't add a pound.

CHAPTER 17

Yoga, the Yoke between Mind, Body and Spirit
By Kelly Metzger

Blessed are the flexible, for they shall not be bent out of shape.
–Unknown Author

The word "yoga" means to yoke or join. Yoga can bring the body into natural alignment to optimize health and wellness. But yoga goes much further than this. The goal of Yoga is to join our mind, body and spirit with the world around us. Yoga teaches mastery over the mind. Traditionally, Yoga refers to Raja Yoga, the ancient science of the mind. The primary text of Raja Yoga is called the "Yoga Sutras of Patanjali." There are almost 200 sutras, traditionally divided into four sections.

First is "Contemplation," most likely given to the student for inspiration to begin the practice. Second is "Practice," practical philosophy and the five basic steps out of the traditional eight limbs of Raja Yoga, along with the benefits, obstacles and ways to overcome the obstacles of the practice. The third is "Accomplishments," a discussion of the final three inner steps of Raja Yoga and an understanding of the powers and accomplishments that come to faithful practitioner. The final section is "Absoluteness," the understanding of Yoga from a cosmic, philosophical viewpoint.

It is still unknown when Patanjali lived or if he was an individual or group of people using this title, but the estimated dates of the Sutras range from 5,000 B.C. to 300 A.D. Patanjali did not "invent" Raja Yoga, rather he systematized and organized the already existing ideas and practices. Thus Patanjali has been considered the "Father of Yoga" and his Sutras are the foundation for all the various forms of meditation and Yoga that exist today.

Yoga can help us realize the spirit of *self*, which is beyond body and mind, beyond personality and ego. A reporter once told a yogi, "I'm interested in the mind-body connection." The mind and body are intimately connected, the yogi replied. "They were both born, and both will die." What will not die is the soul or the higher self. Yoga helps cultivate the realization of the higher self, a seeking to merge our own will with that of the higher self which is Divine or God, whatever suites your religious or spiritual faith.

This ancient practice helps yoke our individual experiences as life with the source of our being or existence, so that we can overcome the illusion of separateness for the source of life. Yoga is not a religion, rather a practice to awaken our connection and identify with the source of life within your own religion or spiritual belief system. In the Western world there is a tendency to separate or fragment things to yield truths. The practice of yoga will help maintain calmness in all experiences in life, by teaching you to become transparent, allowing emotions both happy and sad to flow through you without destroying your peace of mind. Yoga means eternal happiness, bliss, joy and unconditional love. Yoga is who you are in your natural state. Yoga teaches you to know your intensions and motivations, to cultivate spirit of honesty and self-realization.

Yoga is a popular form of physical exercise. Many Westerners are only aware of the physical postures but in the past decades deeper teachings of Yoga have permeated our Western culture. Yogi Bhajan broke with this long-held tradition of silence. A master of Kundalini by the age of 16 (a rare feat), at age 39 and a recent émigré from India, he left behind a lucrative governmental career with the vision of bringing Yoga to the West.

In the turbulent, drug culture of the 60s, Bhajan first reached out to the youth. He recognized their experimentation with drugs and "altered states of consciousness" expressed a deeper desire to experience a holistic, liberating sense of awareness. Soon realizing that pharmaceuticals provided, at best, a cheap imitation to the peaceful, inner euphoria they could get naturally from Kundalini, and at worst, had debilitating physical and mental side effects, young people began flocking to his classes, arriving by the busloads. Soon his teaching centers began springing up across the United States and then throughout the world.

Within the practice of Hatha Yoga emphasis is put on coordinating, synchronizing and uniting our breath with our movements. Hatha is understood as a conjunct of "ha," (sun) and "tha," (moon), so Hatha Yoga can refer to the union of opposites, such as the sun and moon, masculine and feminine, hard and soft, mind and body, right and left, passive and aggressive, known and unknown. Hatha Yoga means union or uniting of opposites.

Yoga reunites all polarities, reconciles opposites and recreates a state of oneness and connectedness with where we originated. Yoga is the joining of the absolute and relative, unlimited and limited, whole and part, infinite and finite, light and dark, stillness and movement, expansion and contraction, masculine and feminine, and being and doing. Yoga creates a state of balance. While practicing Hatha Yoga we are open to the flow of divine love and we are in the flow of grace. The breath (prana) should flow through the body deeply and without strain. The breath is used as a direct feedback to the practitioner. The breath is a tool to work with the mind. The quality of the breath is used as a guide or barometer as to whether we are straining or calm.

Yogis long ago discovered that the breath controls the mind and the mind controls the body. The breath happens to be a direct reflection of the state of our mind: if the breath is bearing calmness, the mind is calm and quiet. The body is a direct manifestation of the mind. The thoughts we have and the experiences we have gone, or are going, through are held and stored in the body in the form of tension. When practicing Hatha Yoga we look to place ourselves in the now, wholly present with the flow of breath. This not only creates a state of deep relaxation, but also allows us to release past experiences and emotions stored in the body.

While in the practice of Yoga, we practice breath control (pranayama: a regulated, even flow of breath) and sense withdrawal. To control the senses we fix the eyes on a set point. These two techniques done together are medicine to your nervous system. Your nervous system will receive fewer messages and will become restored, relaxed and calm. Using a regulated breath and remaining consciously aware of the flow while funneling your energy inward by controlling and relaxing the eyes, will build focus and concentration and help place the mind into a present state (a state of "now"). The moment is pure. This is the technique of Yoga: to continue to bring ourselves into the moment, back to the breath, where no tension occurs.

In the present moment we are able to experience the truth of who we are. This is where healing begins to take place. The practice of Yoga has no goals. The only goal is the journey, the process. The beautiful thing about Yoga as in life is that it happens to be a journey, an exploration, not a destination. Yoga has no goals, there is no destination. Neither is Yoga a competition, sport nor performance, so we are free to express ourselves in our own unique way. Hatha Yoga is a vehicle flowing with grace along this pathway that is infinitely wide and this pathway is the process of self-discovery, self-realization and total oneness with the self (spirituality).

Yoga teaches us about ourselves and about kindness. Yoga teaches us how to become involved and present in our lives, to increase our awareness, broaden our consciousness, eliminate fear and become kinder, happier, more stress-free human beings. And above all else, Yoga is highly enjoyable. Yoga calms and controls the senses and enhances your appreciation of all life. Yoga will enhance the quality of your life if you let it. It is fun and exhilarating. Yoga helps you rise to the challenge of living. It keeps you from being ground down by circumstance. Yoga is known to bring freedom to the body and clarity to the mind and leads the student to balance and wisdom. Yoga is rich in benefits for the body and mind, and it is no surprise that people in the West are now discovering that it makes a lot of sense to practice Yoga for peace and longevity.

A Typical Yoga Workout

The mind-body workout begins at the resting phase which lasts five to ten minutes. The exertion level is low and breathing unusually deep. The primary purpose is to exercise the lungs. By maximizing breathing, the body is prepared for an effortless workout. In this phase, the circulatory system prepares and adjusts for increased demands. The body builds a reserve to avoid oxygen debt and exercise stress.

The coordination of deep-breathing techniques with low exercise levels ensures early removal of systemic waste products including lactic acid which could impair cellular respiration during exercise, and pumps life energy into every cell of the body, preparing it for maximal exertion later in the workout. It also drives oxygen into the smallest and usually dormant alveoli in the lungs and uses optimal lung capacity to allow lower breathing rates and comfort during vigorous exercise.

During the resting phase, the exercise load shouldn't exceed 50 percent of training heart rate (THR). This promotes comfort. Most of us have been taught to exercise between 70 and 80 percent THR. At this higher level, lactic acid build-up is so great muscle function is compromised. The result is an uncomfortable workout. When pushed too far, the body shifts into an anaerobic state which is counterproductive.

The Listening Phase

During the listening phase, you learn to recognize the point at which the body shifts into a state of discomfort (more than 50 percent THR capacity). Labored breathing, a pounding heart or the breakdown of form are clues to slow down.

Strain occurs just before the body reaches the blood lactate threshold. Blood lactate impairs energy production and oxygen transport to the muscles. This can be avoided by training your mind to recognize the point of maximum exercise efficiency. Exercise to the point of discomfort then back off for a period of time. This prepares the body for an even higher level of fitness. Monitor your heart rate to ensure you maintain no more than a 50 percent training capacity. Repeatedly ask the body to go beyond the last level of exertion. If this creates strain, reestablish the comfort zone with a slower pace. In time, your body will accommodate your request for higher performance. Getting to your goal may take a little longer using this technique, but it's better than working in a discomfort zone.

The Performance Phase

The performance phase is the natural extension of the listening phase. Comfort and balance through body and mind coordination take your performance to higher levels. If you lose your personal comfort zone, go back to the listening phase to reestablish it.

The key to maximum integration of mind and body is pace. We are accustomed to high-level exercise. But effortless exercise is the common experience of those performing in the Zone.

A calm, focused mind coordinates the dynamic forces of body movements. The performance phase moves exercise to maximum levels while the brain, heart and breath are composed and calm. Your mind and body are on cruise control at an exercise level you established as your maximum comfort zone in the listening phase.

The Cool-Down

The cool-down begins with five to ten minutes of deep nasal breathing combined with low-level exercise. This ensures the removal of any accumulated blood lactate or other post-exercise circulatory waste products. The removal of waste products speeds rejuvenation and muscle repair, and increases performance levels during subsequent workouts.

Next, five to ten minutes are spent doing the Sun Salute. Due to its counter-posing flexion and extension postures, the Sun Salute is one of the most effective means of gaining flexibility. And the best flexibility gains happen immediately after a workout when the muscles are warm. This exercise also provides a heightened state of neuromuscular integration when practiced five to ten minutes at a time.

Yoga teaches you how to know the language of your body. Language is more than words. It includes a bodily sense of experience. Learn how to be receptive to your body's signals, and make it a self-empowering dialogue.

CHAPTER 18

Massage Therapy
By Mary Marino-Strong

Too often we under estimate the power of a touch, a smile, a kind word, a listening ear, an honest compliment, or the smallest act of caring, all of which have the potential to turn a life around.
—Leo Buscaglia

Massage therapy appears to slow down the heart and relax the body. Rather than causing drowsiness, however, massage actually increases alertness. A number of massage therapies are available. Stressed, over-worked individuals keeping up with families, career, or school often set themselves towards goals with steely determination and don't stop until they have to. This is a pattern in many lives today—a pattern that is reflected in steely muscles and joints, chronic pain, diminished immune systems, and a general state of stress. Over time such problems can turn into physical ailments if not addressed. Fortunately, therapeutic massage is increasingly available. It can relieve pain, release stress and anxiety, and help in the repair and recovery of muscles and joints. It stimulates the body's internal systems to support improved immune function as well as overall health and well-being. Massage is an ancient healing method being proven by modern research.

The amount of research on the benefits of massage grows by leaps and bounds every year and reflects both the wide spectrum of applications for therapeutic massage, as well as its increasing inclusion with other treatment forms. According to recent statistics from the American Massage Therapy Association, the number of hospitals offering massage has increased by more than 33 percent in the past two years. Of those hospitals, 71 percent offer massage for stress relief and comfort, 67 percent for pain management, and 52 percent for cancer patients. Hospitals are also using massage therapy to improve mobility and movement for pregnancy, edema, infant care, pre and post-operative care, hospice, and in conjunction with physical therapy.

Why is massage so important? Biochemists that identified receptor sites, neuropeptides and the communication network between the brain, nerves and other parts of the body, help us understand why massage is effective. Massage typically uses hands-on rubbing, squeezing, pressing and otherwise manipulation of muscle tissue and joints using varying degrees of pressure, with or without joint movement. The skin, the body's largest organ, has over 5 million receptor sites sending signals to the brain. The manipulation of muscles in massage activates this immense communication network, triggering a vast chain reaction from the brain throughout all the systems. It involves millions of cells, glands, hormones and other chemicals, organs, blood and neural pathways. Figuratively speaking, it fires up neurotransmitters like Fourth of July fireworks, or a complex computer network sending up a rocket ship. Unlike computers, the body has the distinct advantage of a self-healing or self-regulating capacity.

The results of this flurry of internal activity are as diverse as the individuals receiving massage. Research has shown benefits such as boosting the immune system; reducing blood pressure in stroke patients; easing post-operative pain; easing alcohol withdrawal symptoms; relief of pain, fatigue, stress, anxiety, nausea and depression in cancer patients; and long-lasting soothing for chronic back pain. In fact, massage is the treatment of choice for back pain, surpassing all other complementary therapies. Muscle spasms and pain in post-heart bypass surgery were reduced in patients treated with massage at the hospital after surgery. Patients were so pleased that 60 percent were willing to pay for treatment themselves.

The efficacy of therapeutic massage is further shown by its ability to improve blood circulation and lymph flow, improve oxygenation, flush cell waste, decrease heart rate and blood pressure, increase body heat and tissue respiration, and reduce excess cortisol, which is produced by very high stress levels. (Excess cortisol destroys the body's killer cells thus diminishing one of the immune system's important lines of defense.) Massage can rebalance excess or inadequate energy flow. It helps pre-term infants gain weight, and affection-deprived infants develop. Ashley Montagu, Ph.D., renowned anthropologist and considered the father of massage, found that stubborn eczema healed when mothers spent time massaging their babies.

In addition to its many direct benefits, massage is being used increasingly in collaboration with movement therapies, chiropractic, osteopathy, physical and occupational therapies, and in dental offices. Chair massage can be found in airports and offices, especially accounting offices at tax time. Massage can help clear and still the mind. Tiffany Fields, M.D. of the Touch Research Institute of Miami University has shown the calculation of math problems take half as long with double the accuracy after nine consecutive days of fifteen-minute chair massage. Therapeutic massage can also be an excellent adjunct to psychotherapy and can help enhance self-image, self-esteem and self-empowerment while helping to release unwanted emotions stored in the body.

Choosing a Type of Massage and a Massage Therapist

Realize that not all forms of massage do all things. That's why you need to find out what is available in your area and ask friends and others whose opinions you trust for recommendations. Professional massage associations can be a source of massage referrals as well. In choosing a massage therapist, be sure to find out whether your state requires a license or certification. They help to maintain education levels and ensure public safety. Be sure your massage therapist displays a current license or certificate; feel free to ask where he or she went to school, what their training was and whether they have specialties. You are the ultimate judge of whether a type of massage or a particular massage therapist is suited to you. Explore a variety of styles and practitioners to make an informed choice, and trust your judgment.

Some Types of Massage:

- **Swedish**, an all-purpose, relaxing massage with long, gliding strokes of variable pressure. It starts lightly and builds to medium or deeper pressure.
- **Deep Tissue, Trigger Point** and **Neuromuscular Therapy** use deep pressure. Typically a deep, or very deep, pressure is applied on a single point at a time and held until the desired muscle release is felt.
- **Asian** massage includes, for example, **Shiatsu, Acupressure, JinShinDo**. These are similar to the

previous category in that deep pressure is applied. They differ in that the pressure is applied to points along a system of meridians to rebalance energy and tone organ systems.

- **Sports Massage** is specifically oriented to athletic performance, muscle and joint recovery. It is muscle-specific and performed using very deep pressure.
- **Myofascial Release (MFR)** technique uses moderate to deep pressure dispersed over a wider area than a single point. It helps to release or unwind deep layers of myofascia that envelop and hold all muscles of the body tightly.
- **Massage and Movement** therapies are less general and more specific to conditions and ailments.
- **Self-Healing Bodywork and Movement Therapy**, pioneered by Meir Schneider, Ph.D., LMT, integrates mind-body resources to address challenging conditions and degenerative ailments. It works with the central nervous system to reprogram ineffective patterns of movement. Schneider says there are over 600 muscles in the body and we typically use only about 50 large, postural muscles. Self-Healing activates use of more muscles in the body while relieving overused muscles. This method tends to have a rhythmic, moderate touch ranging to deep pressure. It is combined with therapeutic movement, visualization, and breathing. It is especially useful with muscular dystrophy, multiple sclerosis, rheumatoid arthritis, Parkinson's, loss of coordination, restricted movement, etc.
- **Reiki, Therapeutic Touch, Touch for Health**, etc. are very gentle. They bring energy to areas that are low, or remove excess energy through the laying on of hands. This can be done directly on the body or above it.
- **Chair Massage** is given while sitting on a massage chair designed to support the head and neck while allowing the rest of the body to be comfortable and accessible to the massage therapist. Usually chair massages are given on-site at a location other than the therapist's office. They are of short duration, from 5 to 15 minutes on average.

What to Expect from a First Massage

If you are receiving massage for the first time, ask your massage therapist what to expect and review the following points with her or him. Your privacy and comfort are important. You should always be draped with a sheet or large towel. A blanket or heater should be available for added warmth, as some people get cool when receiving massage. Only the muscles and joints being massaged should be exposed; private body areas should never be exposed. The massage therapist should leave the room while the client undresses, and the client undresses only to his or her level of comfort. It is perfectly acceptable to leave underwear on during massage. Chair massage is performed fully clothed. Remember, it is your massage; feel free to express your preferences, whether it be regarding the degree of pressure, type of massage oil, temperature, music, or if you prefer more time be given to a sore area such as your back or neck, etc. At the end of an hour's massage, an adept practitioner's clients will likely be wishing they didn't have to get off the massage table. It's good to notice how you feel as the day progresses as it provides feedback for your internal communicators and can deepen the effect of your massage.

CHAPTER 19

The Relaxation Response

If the body sticks around while the brain wanders off, a longer lifetime becomes a burden on self and society. Extending the life of the body gains most meaning when we preserve the life of the mind.

– William Safire

Herbert Benson of Harvard published a landmark book on transcendental meditation (TM) in 1975 called *The Relaxation Response*. The book outlines a simple method for lowering heart rate, decreasing blood pressure, affecting metabolism, and controlling pain. TM is a set of mind-body exercises that counteract and reduce the harmful effects of stress. While practicing TM, the mind and body settle down and experience restful alertness. As the mind becomes more silent, the body becomes deeply relaxed. TM adherents believe that this state contributes to greater creativity, improved learning, better reasoning skills, and increased mental well-being.

A quiet environment and comfortable position are important but not critical to elicit your body's "relaxation response." You'll need a mental device—mantra, prayer or focus on an object—and a passive attitude. After relaxing, visualize a good outcome that you wish to have. Benson drew from Eastern spiritual traditions to create TM. He essentially "secularizes" these traditions to make them more accessible for Westerners.

Practitioners claim that TM correlates with improvements in physical health. These include improved blood pressure and heart rate, better metabolism, and the ability to control pain. Studies are still ongoing to determine the extent to which this and other forms of meditation alter brain function, heart rate, blood flow and immune function. The clinical findings of Harvard's Mind Body Medical Institute when practicing relaxation techniques include:

- Chronic pain patients reduce their physician visits by 36 percent.

- There is approximately a 50 percent reduction in visits to a HMO after a relaxation-response based intervention, which resulted in estimated significant cost savings.
- Eighty percent of hypertensive patients have lowered blood pressure and decreased medications; 16 percent are able to discontinue all of their medications. These results lasted at least three years.
- Open heart surgery patients have fewer post-operative complications.
- One-hundred percent of insomnia patients reported improved sleep and 91 percent either eliminated or reduced sleeping medication use.
- Infertile women have a 42 percent conception rate, a 38 percent take-home baby rate, and decreased levels of depression, anxiety, and anger.
- Women with severe PMS have a 57 percent reduction in physical and psychological symptoms.
- High school students exposed to a relaxation response-based curriculum had significantly increased their self-esteem.
- Inner city middle school students improved grade score, work habits and cooperation, and decreased absences.

Relaxation training also may be enhanced through biofeedback, such as might be obtained by measuring skin resistance, muscle-energy output, or temperature of the hands or feet with a biofeedback device. The initial use of biofeedback is just to let you know how you are responding to changes in thought or position. Later on, it aids in training you to become more relaxed by letting you know which types of activities represent your "getting out of your own way" so that your body automatically relaxes. The key is not to try. (Remember what happens when you try to go to sleep? You are more wide awake. Similarly, if you try to relax, you will become tense.) Instead, allow yourself to become relaxed by focusing your thoughts away from the hectic problems of the day. When the mind is focused, whether through meditation or other repetitive mental activities, the body responds with a dramatic decrease in heart rate, breathing, blood pressure and metabolic rate—the opposite effects of the fight-or-flight response.

CHAPTER 20

Focusing Your Mind's Eye

For me, winning isn't something that happens suddenly on the field when the whistle blows and the crowds roar. Winning is something that builds physically and mentally every day that you train and every night that you dream.
            —Emmitt Smith, American Football Player

Neuroscientists discovered the neural mechanisms for visualization, a common technique used by star athletes, actors, artists, surgeons and performers. The brain influences the body, and the body affects the mind. The brain can simulate body states before they occur or body states that do not occur at all, something called "mirror imaging." Mirror neurons are active when you perform certain tasks, but they also fire when you imagine or watch someone else perform the same specific task.

This technique takes your focus away from your problems. The imaging can take the shape of people, places, or things, or it can involve focusing on bright to calm colors (and back) or bright to calm music (and back). Visualizing an accomplishment, such as climbing a mountain with supportive aid as needed (from family, friends, or spiritual strength), provides a sense of accomplishing a goal and the peace and good feelings that accompany it.

Visualization, creating a picture, movie, or image for yourself, is an excellent way of healing and improving your way of life and reducing stress. Draw a picture, still or moving, of how you would like to look, what relationships you'd like to have, what type of career you'd like to be working in, or how to play your favorite sport.

Visualization has been used in sports for decades, especially by Russians athletes. Jack Nicolas visualizes his next shot in golf three times from beginning to end immediately before every shot. The Russians use it for their weight lifters. I use it before I serve in tennis or before difficult surgeries while I'm washing my hands immediately before entering the operating room. Visualization improves results.

The visualization needs to be realistic, though. At 5'-10" I don't think I could ever dunk a basketball (best I ever did was touch the bottom of the net), but I improved my three-point shot rate by visualizing the complete shot. My foul-shot rate also improved. Visualization works better with increasing results if you do it regularly.

Write down the results you want, say the results you want (affirmation) and use positive statements (invocations). Andre Agassi told himself, "You can't miss." Arnold Palmer said, "I have a great putting gaze." Avoid negative affirmations, such as "You're not good enough" or "Why try." Remember the placebo effect.

Visualization works better if you do it during or after meditations with a consciousness to pure awareness (a focus, directed concentration). The image you visualize can be a still picture, or even a slow moving video in your mind's eye. Practice makes perfect, so do it often. Visual imagery has great value for stress relief or improving your life, including weight loss, smoking cessation and seeking a new career or better job.

Smell it, feel it, hear it. Imagery is a flow of thought you can see, hear, feel, smell or taste. An image is an inner representation of your experience or your fantasies. It is the currency of dreams, memories and future goals, great or small. Your autonomic nervous system doesn't respond to ordinary thoughts like "salivate" or "palpitate" but does respond to imagery, the mind's eye. Imagery is the interface between what we call the body and mind.

CHAPTER 21

Music Makes Good Medicine
By Linda Wright-Bower

Music speaks what cannot be expressed, soothes the mind and gives it rest, heals the heart and makes it whole, flows from heaven to the soul.

—Unknown Author

In 1997, a young boy in Virginia won state and regional honors for his Science Fair project. He discovered that mice treated to regular doses of Mozart were able to navigate a maze 20 minutes faster than mice treated to rock music.[227] Sometimes science corroborates the obvious. Heart rate, blood pressure and breathing rate fluctuate in respond to music, with an arousal effect seen with increasing tempo. Slow, meditative music induces a relaxing effect, especially during the pauses. Research has shown that music can enhance memory and concentration and decrease anxiety and pain perception. Music therapy is cost-effective, enjoyable and has no side effects—it makes good medicine.

Hardly a day goes by that we don't hear music. Music permeates our environment. We hear songs on the radio, jingles on commercials, the chanting and singing of children at play, or popular melodies hummed by people at work. Music is a pervasive phenomenon that most people enjoy. More over, music helps connect us to key values and spiritual concepts such as joy, hope, grace, forgiveness and beauty in addition to evoking thoughts, feelings and changes in physiology.

When Mozart was composing at the end of the eighteenth century, the city of Vienna was so quiet that fire alarms could be given verbally, by a shouting watchman mounted on top of St. Stefan's Cathedral. In twentieth-century society, the noise level is such that it keeps knocking our bodies out of tune and out of their natural rhythms. This ever-increasing assault of sound upon our ears, minds, and bodies adds to the stress load of civilized beings trying to live in a highly complex environment.

The discipline of music therapy has grown substantially throughout the United States and other countries of the world. Music therapy is currently defined as an evidence-based health care profession that includes the prescribed use of music and music activities by a trained professional to address specific non-musical goals. Music therapists assess client strengths and needs, measure behaviors, create goals and objectives, document progress and evaluate progress.

Research in the psychology of music and the music therapy discipline demonstrates the variety of music therapy applications with different age groups, which we could call from the "womb" to the "tomb" and beyond. Music therapists work with many types of medical conditions and mental disorders in a variety of settings including special education, hospital and childbirth, prisons, cancer clinics, hospice and the end of life care. The way the music is used can also be diverse. Music therapists use a variety of instruments and types of music in the music therapy sessions.

Music is used therapeutically in several different ways. The use of musical jingles and musical phrases has been used to teach academic skills to those with autism or other learning challenges and to teach or "reteach" speaking with people who have aphasia. Music, playing or listening, can be used as a reward for appropriate behavior, attention span, and various social skills. Music may serve as a background for learning such as when background music is used to encourage on-task behavior. Music and movement have long been used to assist individuals head support and body control. The physical aspects of the music, specifically rhythm, can "cue" or entrain and result in improved gait or physical movements associated with rehabilitation. Timing and music is also a factor when combining relaxation techniques with music making. It is interesting to note that greater results occur when live music is used with relaxation techniques.

Music therapy includes the use of behavioral, biomedical, developmental, educational, humanistic and adaptive music instruction. It addresses physical, emotional, cognitive and social needs of individuals.

Finally, music and participation in music therapy can serve as a reflection of learned skills and current progress when compared with earlier functioning. A client who was once aggressive now attends music therapy without violent upsets. Another client explores issues of childhood and abuse through songwriting, improvisation, group drumming, and discussion of song lyrics. A nursing home patient becomes less depressed over a period of time when involved in a hymn singing or spirituality music therapy group. Music therapy can treat an array of developmental disorders, including Down syndrome and attention deficit hyperactivity disorder.

Recorded music is also used in some music therapy situations. Music therapists may also record original client songs or compose special pieces for therapeutic purposes, as is often the case in hospice work. In summary, music therapists use music making, such as playing drums or singing to assist clients in making positive changes in their health status. Other popular techniques include musical games, music and dance, music and movement, music-based relaxation, music discussion, songwriting, music and arts, therapeutic music instruction, and group music making or improvisation.

Common to the work of all music therapists is the use of client preferred music. It is important to note that while music is universal it is not a "language." Music tends to be regarded as sedative if it has melodic melodies, even rhythms, and a tempo slower than one's heart beat. Uplifting or energizing music tends to have tempos slightly faster than one's heart beat, use of syncopated rhythms and certain kinds of instrumentation. However, everyone's responses to music are unique. Not everyone will react the same way to a song such as Bobby McFerrin's "Don't Worry, Be Happy" song. Some will like it, others will hate it.

Original or newly composed music might be more appropriate for tasks such as gait training, music-based exercise and some music and relaxation techniques. The scientific use of rhythm-based techniques is an emerging field within music therapy called "neurological music therapy." This school of music therapy focuses on the brain's physiological responses to rhythm for the neurological improvement of gait, language, movement, executive functioning skills, and attention. This science-based model of music therapy treatment involves a shift in emphasis from music therapy as a social science to music therapy as a neuroscience. Neurological music therapy has been applied to individuals with Parkinson's Disease, aphasia, stroke rehabilitation and other conditions associated with traumatic brain injury. Researchers are also exploring applications with the autism spectrum and other developmental disabilities.

Some people surround themselves with music, or work in a music permeated atmosphere. Worship often starts with music, as do other social and community group meetings. Many forms of exercise involve physical routines choreographed to music. Pep band music and chants are a common part of many team sports. Advertisers use music to sell products. Companies count on people to recognize musical jingles and songs related to their products. Shopping facilities play music in the background, as do restaurants. The proliferation of affordable electronic devices such as the i-Pod makes it easy for people to collect and use their favorite music in a variety of settings. Listening to music is one of the most popular coping skills used to deal with stress.

Physiologically speaking, music requires use of your entire brain. The left side of the brain is responsible for identifying familiar tunes, recognizing rhythm patterns as well as analyzing form and structure associated with music. The right brain processes implied harmonic relations (chord patterns), imagery, pitch judgments, the "big picture" or gestalt of the piece in addition to cognitions and overtones. So if you sing a familiar tune you need the left brain to recognize the tune and the right brain to produce it. Thus, music can be used to shape the neural mappings in your brain.

The music can also affect your automatic nervous system. For example, people exhibit a stronger hand grip when listening to marches than they do for lullabies. Music can affect your breathing, blood pressure and skin temperature, too. Even people who are deaf respond to the vibrations of musical sound.

There a number of ways to use music to address cognitive and mental stimulation needs. Research demonstrates that people who keep mentally active are at a lower risk of developing degenerative conditions like Alzheimer's disease. Mental stimulation can be addressed by learning more about music, such as taking a music appreciation class, learning to play an instrument, playing music singing with others, playing musical games, journaling to music, and meditating to music.

Just as it is important to put healthy foods in your body, it is also important to consider the lyrics when listening to music. Lyrics that promote violence, bigotry, hatred, and crime are negative conditioning that should be avoided. Parents have a responsibility to help children learn to pick music and lyrics which reflect the values of the family. It is important to note that children begin to prefer rock music over folk and traditional children's music as early as the first and second grade. Let the musical lyrics be health-enhancing.

Since music is known to tap the emotions, it would make sense to use music as an accompaniment to celebrations and ceremonies that we want to remember. We might end our day by listening to calming music, or begin our day with the alarm clock set to our favorite music station. While driving to a job interview we might listen to energizing music or music with positive messages in the lyrics. If we are nervous about the job interview, we might be better off to listen to calming music, recite affirmations or practice breathing slowly. But never listen to music and relaxation imagery recordings while you are driving. Your body and your passengers need your focus behind the wheel.

Music as Catharsis

One of the healthiest things we can do is to allow ourselves to feel the feelings we have despite being told to "get over it." Nothing is more maddening than being told, through words or deeds, that our feelings don't matter. One of my clients found that few people wanted to listen to feelings related to her pregnancy loss. Her means of honoring her grief included reading poems written by mothers who had lost a fetus or neonate, journaling to music and improvising lyrics while actively playing new age music on the piano. She poured her heart out in song during those dark moments and eventually felt better. Listening or writing to music is one way to experience and honor one's grief in a private manner. What better way to comfort our hurting than to do it for ourselves.

Songs and hymns support us when we are grieving and help connect us to memories of the past. Hospice music therapists know the value of using music from the young adult years to explore a patient's life and meaningful relationships. Hearing one's favorite love songs from courtship can renew feelings associated with falling in love, even if only for a few moments. In general, research shows that people prefer music from their young adult years. This is especially helpful information when selecting music for patients who might have memory or language impairments due to Alzheimer's disease or dementia.

One way to use music in a healthy way is to rewrite the lyrics of a favorite or meaningful song. In this way, one can personalize the events of the song and allow for individual expression of feelings, which might be otherwise difficult to verbalize. Another method would be to play a musical instrument, preferable after a period of musical instruction, in a manner associated with feelings in the here and now. For example, if I'm in a joyful mood, I might choose to play "Amazing Grace" in an upbeat, peppy manner. While I would do for myself, it might not be appropriate for professional use with others. It might also be good to build a music listening repertoire of "feel good" songs, a kind of emotional music-based first-aid kit that you can access when you want to elevate your mood. Maybe you find that you feel better when given some time to listen to the Beach Boys or Dixie Chicks. For another person, dance music and music from the Big Band era work best.

Religious music or hymn singing may provide a calming and peaceful death. Many music therapists play music, carefully matching the tempo of the music to the patient's breathing rate, as a patient actively dies. Again, it is important to know the music preferences of the patient because he or she may have specific wishes. Perhaps a person will want to hear the Beatles or Fleetwood Mac as they move on.

Matching Moods with Music

Elizabeth J. Miles, an ethnomusicologist and author, compiled numerous musical selections for six specific emotional states—relax, focus, uplift, create, cleanse, heal and energize—and recommends classical music for each. She shows you how to use music as a mood-enhancement tool—finding just the right sounds to help you handle anxiety, enhance your creativity, boost your IQ, control pain, get motivated, have better sex and more.

A "psychomusicologist" who provides an extensive music listening reference listing along with specific exercises is John Ortiz, M.D., author of *The Tao of Music*. Ortiz provides over 24 musical menus that include a variety of styles of music such as Jazz and popular music selections. For example, six pages are devoted to music selections that people can use to enhance romance. He includes specific music exercises for exploring stress, anger, pain, sleep problems, aging, grief, procrastination, communication, relationships, letting go, creativity and other listening suggestions. Exercises also include other healthy practices commonly addressed in mind-body publications such as affirmations, breath work, thought stopping, chanting, toning, and mantric sounds.

Chuck Lange created a number of DVD selections that include both music and visual scenes. These are helpful for those who find that they return to stressful or work-related thoughts when listening to music. "Tropical Rhythms" and "First Snows of Christmas" are two examples that combine nature images with relaxing sounds of guitar and keyboard.

The use of music in physical exercise programs is commonplace in our society. Seeing a jogger with headphones is a daily occurrence. Video workout tapes include music selections where tempos are carefully manipulated according to the physical demands of the exercise. Yoga programs, in the community or commercial CD programs often include mysterious-sounding music with an Eastern bent. Many of us are already involved in using music in a healthy way as we exercise.

Two additional ways to use healthy music for physical body enhancement are breath work and pain management. One popular relaxation strategy includes slow breathing. By slowing down the breath anxiety lessens and results in a greater intake of oxygen, further promoting the mind and body relaxation response. You may not have an hour to listen to a relaxation tape, but just five minutes of slow breathing to music can be an aid in promoting focus and reducing tension.

Music can also be used to manage pain. Music, often paired with verbal imagery suggestions, allows our brain to focus on the musical elements and words, thus giving our mind the perception of reduced pain. The gate theory of pain implies that the brain becomes absorbed in processing aural cues and thus has less room to focus on pain. In essence, the music functions as a diversion or distraction stimulus. Research has shown that children are more cooperative and experience less pain when doctors play music during invasive medical procedures.

Music can also be a distraction stimulus during childbirth. Music can be selected to accompany various stages of labor. The music needs to be carefully chosen to support recommended breathing suggestions given in childbirth classes. Some parents may want to create a special "birthing" recording that includes celebration-type music to be played at the actual moment of birth. Music can also be used by the mother during breast feeding to provide a soothing atmosphere, enhance a mother's ability to relax, and promote longer feedings. Furthermore, musical pacifiers have been used to promote nutritive sucking in premature neonates.

Imagery is often supported and enhanced through the use of music. One creative imagery practitioner and author who has used music extensively is Belleruth Naparstek. She's the voice on the majority of the CDs that her company produces. The Health Journeys Company sells recordings of imagery and music for various conditions such as losing weight, managing the symptoms of cancer, reducing stress, improving surgery outcomes, and reducing anxiety. The music is composed specifically for these recordings and is a new age type. Thus, consumers should have no conscious associations, positive or negative, to the music. The novelty of the music allows the listener to focus on the imagery script without interfering memories evoked by familiar music.

Some of the lesser known or unconventional uses of music, such as sound healing and vibration, along with such practices as chanting, charka meditation and drumming can be found in *Mind Body Spirit Workbook: A Handbook of Health*.

Perhaps the most important way to use healthy music is in the promotion of spiritual practices. Simply put, spirituality is the pursuit of the divine or the ability to see the sacred in everyday life. *Spiritual Rx* is a book of quotes, readings, imagery scripts, art and music references, poems, and activity suggestions for over 26 spiritual practices, such as kindness and forgiveness.

There a number of ways to use healthy music in the pursuit of spirituality. One way is to recognize when a piece of music evokes a feeling of peace, contentment or joy in living. Another is to select relaxing music to listen to while you read books related to spirituality. People can write poetry to spiritual music or write about spiritual topics such as patience. Using gentle music to accompany meals, bathing and other rituals can assist a person in staying present and being mindful.

One might explore the meaning of spiritual concepts through a spiritual drumming workshop or other drumming circle event. Yet another way is to take a book such as *Spiritual Rx* and devote a week to practicing that attribute. For example, if I were to select "attention" for the week I might listen to some of the suggested pieces of music, use the imagery script during meditation to music, journal about some of the spiritual quotations in the book, and watch movies associated with that particular practice. One could also spend a month studying a particular spiritual practice such as "teachers" and use sections of that chapter to spark personal growth writings, readings or interactions.

Making music and using music allows us to be connected to the larger world we call our universe. Furthermore, making music often involves a number of people or a musician and an accompanist. Using music in worship is usually carried out in a community church or synagogue. Discussing music, the lyrics, and the use of music in movies often occurs in spoken or written conversation. Listening to live music allows people to feel connected to the musicians and the soul of their talent and inspiration.

Healthy opportunities for using music in healthy ways exist whether you are a music amateur or music consumer. You might want to start a music listening group at your local bookstore where people could come once a month to discuss various songs, pieces of music, and listen to speakers. Many of these bookstores include coffee bars and cafes, which would add to the relaxing atmosphere for such a group. The Lowery Organ Company sponsors group organ lessons for seniors and also include wellness exercises. Results have been dramatic, especially when compared to the health benefits of seniors taking individual lessons.

You do not have to be a music therapist or patient to enjoy the benefits of therapeutic music, recreational music making and music wellness programs. It is appropriate to call any personal use of music for health purposes "therapeutic." Inclusion of music in your health practice allows one to deepen and reinforce the mind-body connection path to better health. Exercise good judgment in selecting music lyrics and listen to your heart when determining the health value of specific selections. Sometimes when we're in pain, medications can only go so far. Music is a versatile health-care intervention. "There is no feeling, except the extremes of fear and grief that does not find relief in music," said George Eliot.

CHAPTER 22

A Dose of Laughter
By Kevin Lee Smith

The human race only one really effective weapon and that is laughter.
–Mark Twain

The belief that laughter is the best medicine has been around for ages. Throughout history, many have considered that there are beneficial effects from joy, humor, and laughter. Greek philosophers, including Plato and Aristotle, wrote treatises on humor. In 1790 the German philosopher Immanuel Kant described the physical effects of humor and defined humor as a talent that enabled one to look at things from a different perspective. In medieval physiology science, the definition of humor was "moisture" or "vapor." If you recall from Chapter 2, humor referred to the four principal fluids of the body: blood, phlegm, choler (yellow bile), and melancholy (black bile). A proper balance of the four was called good humor, and a preponderance of any one constituted ill humor.

The notion that humor and laughter can improve our ability to cope with difficulties and to stay healthy continues to be a popular concept. Interest in this area has increased significantly since Norman Cousins' account of the role of laughter in his recovery from a painful collagen disorder that he presented in his popular book, *Anatomy of an Illness*. Interest and continued scientific study continues in this area, as we have witnessed a growing acceptance of looking at mind-body connections to our health along with complementary and alternative health therapies.

Nurse and humor expert Vera Robinson described the phenomenon of humor as "any communication which is perceived by any of the interacting parties as humorous and leads to laughing, smiling or a feeling of amusement."[228] A dictionary definition describes humor as "the quality of being laughable or comical," and "the ability to perceive, enjoy, or express what is comical or funny." Humor can be the process of either producing or perceiving the comical. Humor varies among individuals. However, there are predictable stimuli for laughter and usual responses.

Defining humor as merely "being funny" would be misguided. Sharing humor is not about *being* funny. You do not need to be a stand-up comedian or wear a red clown nose and big shoes to share humor. You simply need to be open to sharing spontaneous humor and joy when the situation is suitable. Focusing on the *sense* aspect of humor relates to your ability to perceive, appreciate and respond to the multitude of humorous possibilities around us.

A relatively new term has emerged, "Therapeutic Humor," which refers to the intentional use of humor by a health care professional or other care provider, teacher, or others. The Association for Applied and Therapeutic Humor (2006) defines therapeutic humor as follows:

> Any intervention that promotes health and wellness by stimulating a playful discovery, expression, or appreciation of the absurdity or incongruity of life's situations. This intervention may enhance work performance, support learning, improve health, or be used as a complementary treatment of illness to facilitate healing or coping, whether physical, emotional, cognitive, social, or spiritual.

Most of the humor that is employed on a daily basis is of the spontaneous type—situational humor that arises out of the normal absurdities of the day's activities. This type of humor is also a very effective communication tool when used to break the ice with clients, co-workers, and others. An attempt is made to lighten up the situation; this is a sign of caring and interest and allows for a free exchange of thoughts, feelings and emotions. "Life does not cease to by funny when someone dies, anymore than it ceases to be serious when someone laughs," said George Bernard Shaw.

The Science of Laughter

Laughter creates a cascade of physiological changes in the body. Scientists studied the effects of mirthful laughter on heart rate and on the oxygen saturation level of peripheral blood and respiratory phenomena. In contrast to other emotions, laughter involves extensive physical activity. It increases respiratory activity and oxygen exchange, increases muscular activity and heart rate, and stimulates the cardiovascular system, the sympathetic nervous system, and the production of catecholamines, sometimes referred to as "feel good hormones." The actual measurement of endorphin production related to laughter does not have a strong scientific basis, but there is ongoing research in this area.

The relaxation state follows the laughter state in which respiration rate, heart rate, and muscle tension return to normal. Blood pressure lowers and a state exists similar to the impact of hearty exercise. Other studies have found that humor and laughter increase levels of immune factors in the body.

Loma Linda University humor researcher Lee Berk and colleagues demonstrated that laughter lowered serum cortisol levels, or stress hormones, increased the amount of infection fighting activated T-lymphocytes, and increased the number and activity of natural killer cells. The changes were sustained over a twelve hour period. Laughter is good medicine.

Another research study assigned hundreds of heart-attack survivors to one of two groups. The control group received standard advice regarding medications, diet, and exercise. The treatment group received additional counseling on relaxation, smiling, laughing at themselves, admitting mistakes, taking time to enjoy life, and renewing their religious faith. Over three years, the treatment group experienced half as many repeat heart attacks as the control group.

In a pediatric oncology setting, nurses and researchers found a direct relationship with a high sense of humor and psychosocial adjustment to cancer as well as fewer incidences of infection among children with high coping humor scores.

Humor as Catharsis

Humor has been considered an adaptive coping mechanism. Freud regarded humor and laughter as one of the few socially acceptable means for releasing pent-up frustrations and anger, a cathartic mechanism for preserving psychic or emotional energy. Humor and laughter alter our perspective in various situations. Laughter can counteract negative emotions; it allows people to transcend predicaments, conquer painful circumstances, and cope with difficulties. By focusing energy elsewhere, humor can diffuse the stress of difficult events. The use of humor even has been shown to reduce threat-induced anxiety.

Research has suggested that there is a possible link between happiness and long life. In a study of the sisters of Notre Dame, the diaries of the nuns, who joined back in the 1930s, were examined. Researchers studied the diary entries and counted the number of times they used positive and negative words. Some entries were quite joyful while others were gloomy. Researchers divided the group into "happy nuns" and "not so happy nuns." Once they joined the order, their lives were approximately the same including diet, type of work, and daily routine. However, the life expectancy was not the same. In the less positive nuns group, two thirds died before their eighty-fifth birthday. In the happy nuns group, 90 percent were still alive. The happiest nuns lived approximately nine years longer than the least happy nuns.

Your Own Humor Profile

When evaluating your own sense of humor, you should consider what type of humor seems most natural. Consider preferences for spontaneous versus formal humor. The comfort levels of the individual and the recipient of humor should also be considered. Like all skills, you can always work on improving your sense of humor. The first and biggest barrier to using humor is the fear of appearing foolish or of losing control over one's self-image. Humor that is divisive in any way should be avoided. Spontaneous comments on a neutral topic such as the weather, the setting, or yourself can help you to see if the individual is open to humor, though readiness for humor may or may not be apparent.

Any attempt to come up with a one-size-fits-all approach to humor would be doomed to fail. There are a multitude of variables and dynamics that determine whether your attempt at humor is a hit or is dead on arrival. Individual characteristics, personality, and demeanor are complex making it nearly impossible to replicate another's approach to humor. One physician I know has a teddy bear on his stethoscope and occasionally pulls out a miniature harmonica as playful distraction for his pediatric patients. Another physician (whose physical appearance would lead one to believe that he could fit into the old joke "he initially wanted to be an accountant, but he didn't have the personality") has a straight face and a dry wit; most of the time his humor works. Perhaps the incongruity of how he appears and what he says adds to his humor. There is no one-size fits all approach to humor, but basic guidelines are helpful.

Recommended low risk humor styles include self-deprecating humor, puns and plays on words, or a playful greeting. The most important factors in using humor is to be genuine, keep it simple, keep it somewhat relevant, and if in doubt—leave it out. If the other person initiates the humor, do your best to go along with them.

The timing of the use of humor is crucial to its success. What may be funny to a person in one situation may not seem funny at another time. Humor and laughter are inappropriate at the height of a crisis, although it can be useful to allay tension as the crisis subsides. Inside jokes among friends or colleagues can seem offensive or callous to outsiders who may overhear them. Laughing at others negates confidence and damages teamwork, whereas laughing *with* others builds confidence, brings people together, and pokes fun at our common dilemmas. Sometimes aggressive remarks are made under the pretext of joking, whereas this may be a type of masked aggressive verbal behavior.

The use of humor has been and will continue to be an important aspect of our lives and is a worthy topic of continued study. Being aware of the importance of humor is an essential starting point. Individuals can use this information to incorporate humor into their lives to make their work and personal lives more enjoyable and to become more effective in their endeavors. Perhaps this "best medicine" can add years or healthier years to your life. Even if it does not, there are few known risks of using humor and laughter, unless you just had an appendectomy.

CONCLUSION

All of life is a coming home. Salesmen, secretaries, coal miners,
beekeepers, sword swallowers, all of us. All the restless hearts of the
world, all trying to find a way home.

—Hunter "Patch" Adams

In the early 1990s, the White House and Congress became mired in the political process of how to improve our health care system. What we heard from Washington talking heads, op-ed writers and focus groups was that despite all the advanced technology and soaring costs, key US health indicators such as life expectancy and infant mortality rates were lagging behind other industrialized countries and millions of Americans were uninsured. The problems are the same today, only worse. After not wanting to touch health care reform in the post-Clinton era, politicians know that health care needs reform. The trillion dollar question isn't how the crisis came about, but how—according to what codes, values and customs—it will change. The real battles are internal, and they turn on the character of the society and culture being forged.

For those many doctors now burning out from the challenges of modern medical practice, mind-body medicine offers hope. Doctors can find greater satisfaction and meaning from work by connecting with patients in deeper and more rewarding ways. Mind-body medicine offers proven approaches using the patient's own inner resources. Physicians can draw from the spiritual dimension that acknowledges what our patients have been telling us all along. They want more from us as healers than purely a physical approach. They want us to share our hearts, souls, minds, and, yes, our prayers with theirs in a collaborative process of healing.

What's learned that beyond the might of our most sophisticated medical equipment is a physician's humanity—the listening ear, the healing touch, the power of the word. Physicians have considerable influence, presumably derived from their medical expertise. Patients often regard their recommendations as authoritative. For the ill, doctors stand for hope. Patients can be helped by the best of mind-body medicine such as yoga and meditation as well as good nutrition, exercise and support groups. The destructive effect of stress and overwork require new treatments.

Cultivating holistic health by considering the patient's mental, emotional and social needs fosters harmony, and therefore health within the person, family, and community. The road less traveled in our culture is the acknowledgment that life is suffering, and the pursuit of wellness—physical, intellectual, emotional and spiritual—through discipline or what the great American author, poet and philosopher Ralph Waldo Emerson called "self-reliance" of the mind.

The classic book, *The Road Less Traveled*, recommends certain tools for experiencing the pain of problems constructively. The same techniques can be applied to managing your health: delaying gratification, acceptance of responsibility and balancing. Developing the *will* to use these simple tools is the first step towards lasting wellness. In an age of uncertainty, Western medicine can appear to provide concrete answers. And the faith that medicine can eventually cure most diseases illuminates one of our most basic hopes: to live forever. Doctors must have the patient's best interest at heart. In turn, the patient must be more than the passive recipient. Doctors acknowledge the role that patients can and should play in their own healing when they pay attention to their patient's emotions, beliefs and ways of handling stress.

We wrote this book to reconnect the doctor to the patient, the patient to the community and the brain to the body. Half of patients seeking medical care have pain or illness that could be diagnosed and treated without expensive tests or heroic interventions such as surgery. Health care providers and patients need to know the latest scientific research proving the brain's influence on the body, and the body on the brain. In a country dedicated even more than most to individualism, it is difficult to imagine efforts and resources for health care reform by government without the commitment of the people. Ultimately, the health of Americans depends not on what others do for them, but on what they are willing to do for themselves.

ACKNOWLEDGMENTS

As Esther Sternberg duly noted in her book, *The Balance Within*, "Whenever a new field comes into being, it comes up against the older dogmas." And so the idea for this book came up against some odd resistance from "old school" physicians who were unfamiliar with the new science behind brain-immune or "mind-body" connections. It is our sincere hope that the substantial scientific evidence cited in our book will help change the way physicians and surgeons practice medicine. If the doctors won't change, the patients will lead them to the water.

Several people inspired, supported or contributed to this book including the dynamic and inspirational co-founder of the Kachmann Mind Body Institute, Kelly Metzger. Thank you to our hard-working and talented graphics designer, Justin Bays for the beautiful book cover. The creative Terry Ratliff and Wayne Schaltenbrand of Rat Art produced the bold illustrations. A long-time friend and tennis partner, John Crawford, M.D. read the manuscript and gave brilliant feedback. (See you on the court, John). My eldest son, Jeffrey Kachmann, M.D. offered his wise insights as a fellow neurosurgeon; and my youngest daughter, Heidi Kachmann Anderson lent her talented editorial eye. Our editor, Dawn Josephson of Cameo Publications helped copy edit and organize the book with her excellent editorial focus.

Karl Engelman, M.D., former professor and director of Cardiovascular Medicine at the University of Pennsylvania, read part of the manuscript and provided his tenured insight and words of caution. Gene Landrum, M.D., friend, author and creative genius contributed to the section on "Creative Visualization." We were also fortunate to have one of the country's best chiropractors, James M. Cox drafted the section on "Chiropractic: The Healing Touch." British pain specialist, Richard Walker, M.D. graciously contrasted the differing outcomes of patients with chronic pain in our chapter on "The Pain Enigma."

Award-winning music therapist, Linda Maurine Wright-Bower wrote the section in the book on music therapy. Linda earned advanced music therapy certification from the Robert Unkefer

Academy for Neurologic Music Therapy at Colorado State University. She is a prolific workshop teacher in the areas of music therapy, gerontology, mental health, as well as college teaching, supervision and curriculum development. Linda has implemented the healing power of music therapy in various areas of critical care, including hospice, oncology and neurology.

Thank you to tai chi and qigong expert, Debrah Roemisch for her contributions to the section on Eastern healing. Mary Marino-Strong of Joint Ventures in Health drafted the healing section in the book on massage. And Kevin Lee Smith of the University of Minnesota, School of Nursing created the section in this book on humor and health.

Thanks to the bright entrepreneur and dedicated businessman, Peter Boebeck of Mitchell's Book Store for his outstanding support of the community. Vince Robinson, editor and part-owner of *INK* newspaper also deserves our gratitude for his gracious support. To Nicholas Dawidoff—brilliant craftsman, kind and gentle critic—and the students of Provincetown Arts Center: thank you for getting us started early in the game. And to Amy Bloom—see you in P-town? And last but never least, to the eternal everyman Daedalus: *il sogno delle vite dell'Italia!*

Most of all, Dr. Kachmann would like to thank his beloved patients who inspire him daily. You make all the difference. Nor could we have spent the long hours researching, emailing, talking on cell phones in two different states, writing, editing, and rewriting this book without the inspiration, love and patience of our soul mates and creative soundboards, Rhonda Kachmann and Scott Geltz. To Kim's children Jessica, Samantha and Coulson—mommy adores you. And to Carolyn Kachmann, thank you for believing in us from the beginning. Al Dios: todo. See you at the Kachmann Mind-Body Institute: http://www.kachmannmindbody.com/.

REFERENCES

Introduction

1. Smith, R., "Primary Care Clinicians Treat Patients with Medically Unexplained Symptoms: A Randomized Controlled Trial," *Journal of General Internal Medicine*, 21: 7, p. 671, July 2006.
2. Damasio, A., <u>Descartes Error</u>, Avon Books, 1994.
3. Beck, A., "The Flexner Report and the Standardization of American Medical Education," Journal of the American Medical Association, 291:2139-2140; 2004.
4. Pert, C., <u>Molecules of Emotion</u>, Scribner, 1997.
5. Ibid, Kandel, E.
6. Thernstrom, M., "My Pain, My Brain," *The New York Times*, May 14, 2006.
7. Smith, R., "Primary Care Clinicians Treat Patients with Medically Unexplained Symptoms: A Randomized Controlled Trial," *Journal of General Internal Medicine*, 21: 7, p. 671, July 2006.
8. Seaward, B., <u>Essentials of Managing Stress</u>, Jones and Bartlett Publishers, 2006.
9. Kawachi, I., "A Prospective Study of Anger and Coronary Heart Disease: The Normative Aging Study," *Circulation*; 94: 2090 – 2095; November 1996.
10. Levine, D., "Anger, Hostility And Depressive Symptoms Linked To High C-Reactive Protein Levels," Duke Med News Release, September 22, 2004.
11. Miller, M., "University of Maryland School of Medicine Study Shows Laughter Helps Blood Vessels Function Better, Scientific Session of the American College of Cardiology," March 7, 2005.
12. Albert, C., et al., "Phobic Anxiety and Risk of Coronary Heart Disease and Sudden Cardiac Death Among Women," *Circulation*, 111:480-487, 2005.
13. National Center for Health Statistics, 2006.
14. Hróbjartsson A, et al, "Is the placebo powerless? An analysis of clinical trials comparing placebo with no treatment," *New England Journal of Medicine*;344:1594-602, 2001.
15. "Yoga and back pain," *Annals of Internal Medicine*, 143:12, p. 849-856, December 20, 2005.
16. Nagourney, E., "Treatments: Acupuncture Fares Well in Headache Experiment," *The New York Times*, August 16, 2005.
17. Bakalar, N., "High Blood Pressure? Meditation May Help," *The New York Times*, June 13, 2006.

Chapter 1

18. Starfield, B., "Is US Health Really the Best in the World?" *Journal of American Medical Association*, 284:483-485; 2000.
19. Abramson, J., <u>Overdosed America</u>, Harper Perennial, 2005.
20. Cousins, N., <u>Anatomy of an Illness</u>, WW Norton & Co.,1979.
21. Centers for Disease Control, "Health, United States," 2004.
22. Cowan, C., Centers for Medicare and Medicaid Services (CMS), Annual Report on Health Care Spending, 2005.
23. Abramson, John, <u>Overdosed America</u>, p. xvii, Harper Perennial, 2005.
24. Abramson, John, "Information Is the Best Medicine," *The New York Times*, September 18, 2004.
25. Brennan T., et al., "Health Industry Practices That Create Conflicts of Interest: A Policy Proposal for Academic Medical Centers," *Journal of American Medical Association*, 284, 295: 429 – 433; 2006.
26. Kolata, G., "Reversing Trend, Big Drop Is Seen in Breast Cancer," *The New York Times*, December 15, 2006.
27. Ibid, Starfield, B.
28. Murray CJL, et al. "Eight Americas: Investigating Mortality Disparities across Races, Counties, and Race-Counties in the United States," *PLoS Medicine*, Vol. 3, No. 9, September 12, 2006.
29. Centers for Disease Control, "Overweight and Obesity Economic Consequences."
30. "Who Is at Greatest Risk for Receiving Poor-Quality Health Care?" *New England Journal of Medicine* 354:1147-1156, 2006.
31. Complementary and Alternative Medicine (CAM) Use Among Adults: United States, 2002. Advance Data No. 343, 20 pp. (PHS) 2004-1250.
32. Kirpatrick, D., et al., "Use of hand-carried ultrasound devices to augment the accuracy of medical student bedside cardiac diagnoses," *Journal of the American Society of Echocardiography*, 18:3, March 2005.
33. Armstrong, D., "Own Image: MRI & CT Centers Offer Doctors Way to Profit on Scans," <u>The Wall Street Journal</u>, May 2, 2005.

34. Iglehart, J., "The New Era of Medical Imaging – Progress and Pitfalls," *The New England Journal of Medicine*, 354:2822-2828, June 29, 2006.
35. Armstrong, D., "Own Image: MRI and CT Centers Offer Doctors Way to Profit on Scans," *The Wall Street Journal*, May 2, 2005.
36. Barlett, D., Steele, J. Critical Condition, Doubleday, 2004.
37. National Center for Health Statistics, Health Insurance Coverage, US Dept. of Health and Human Services.
38. Benson, H., Timeless Healing, Simon & Shuster, 1997.
39. National Center for Complimentary and Alternative Medicine, NCCAM, National Institutes of Health, 2006.
40. Complementary and Alternative Medicine (CAM) Web site.
41. Ibid, Complementary and Alternative Medicine (CAM) Web site.

Chapter 2
42. Ibid, Nuland, S., How We Live.
43. Hippocrates, *On the Sacred Disease*, 400 BC.
44. Nuland, S., *Doctors*, Vintage Books, 1988.
45. Ibid, Hippocrates.
46. Jackson, S., Care of the Psyche, Yale University Press, 1999.
47. Aristotle, *The Nicomachean Ethics*, Book II, 350 B.C.E.
48. Ibid, Jackson, S.
49. Bendick, J., Galen and the Gateway to Medicine, Bethelem Books, 2002.
50. Ibid, Nuland, S., Doctors.
51. Harrington, A. and Brown, T., "Emotions and Disease," Natl. Library of Medicine Exhibit, History of Medicine, 1996.
52. Sontag, S., Illness as Metaphor and AIDS and Its Metaphors, Picador Press, 1989.
53. Ezzati, M., "Causes of cancer in the world: comparative risk assessment of nine behavioral and environmental risk factors," *The Lancet*, Vol. 366, November 19, 2005.
54. Paul, Letter to the Romans, 7:15, New International Version (NIV) Bible, The Gospel Society, 2006.
55. *The Catholic Encyclopedia*, Volume II, Robert Appleton Company, 1907.
56. Ob cit, Jackson, S.
57. Ariel Bar-Sela, Hebbel E. Hoff and Elias Farus, "Moses Maimonides' Two Treatises on the Regimen of Health," *Transactions of the American Philosophical Society*, 1964.

Chapter 3
58. Sternberg, E., *The Balance Within*, W.W. Freeman, 2001.
59. Sontag, S., Illness as Metaphor and AIDS and Its Metaphors, Picador Press, 1989.
60. Ob cit, Nuland, S., Doctors.
61. Erwin H. Ackerknecht, "The History of Psychosomatic Medicine," *Psychological Medicine*, 12, 1982.
62. Arendt, H., The Human Condition, The University of Chicago Press, 1958.
63. Wertheim, M., Pythagoras' Trousers, W. W. Norton & Company, 1997.
64. Bammé, A., Getzinger, G., Wieser, B., "The Mind-Body Problem," Institute for Advanced Studies on Science Technology, Graz Austria.
65. Descartes, R., *Discourse on Method*, in *Discourse on Method and Meditations*, Laurence J. Lafleur, Ed., and Trans., 1960.
66. Jacobs, B., et al., Essays on Kant's Anthropology, Cambridge University Press, 2003.
67. McCormick, M., *Immanuel Kant (1724-1804) Metaphysics, The Internet Encyclopedia of Philosophy*, 2001.
68. Damasio, A. and H., "Minding the Body," *Daedalus*, American Academy of Arts & Sciences, Summer 2006.
69. Ibid, Damasio, A., Descartes Error.
70. Thoreau, H.D., Henry David Thoreau : Collected Essays and Poems, Library of America, 2001.
71. Ibid, Wertheim, M.
72. Darwin, C., *The Descent of Man, and Selection in Relation to Sex*, Princeton University Press, 1981.
73. Ibid, Darwin.
74. Brizendine, L., The Female Brain, Morgan Road Books, 2006.
75. Boydston, J., Home and Work: Housework, Wages, and the Ideology of Labor in the Early Republic, Oxford Univ. Press, 1994.
76. Kinetz, E., "Is Hysteria Real? Brain Images Say Yes," *The New York Times*, September 26, 2006.
77. Maines, R., The Technology of Orgasm: 'Hysteria,' the Vibrator, and Women's Sexual Satisfaction, Baltimore, M.D.: The Johns Hopkins University Press, 1999.
78. Lovering, J., S. Weir Mitchell, New York, NY: Twayne Publishers, Inc., 1971.
79. Freud, E., The Letters of Sigmund Freud, Basic Books, 1975.
80. Jackson, S., Care of the Psyche, Yale University Press, 1999.
81. Gazzaniga, M., The Mind's Past, University of California Press, 2000.

82. Ibid, Damasio, A., <u>The Feeling of What Happens</u>.

83. Angus, D., <u>The Best Short Stories of the Modern Age</u>, Fawcett Books, 1962.

84. Seaward, B., <u>Essentials of Managing Stress</u>, Jones and Bartlett Publishers, 2006.

85. Rosenkranz, M., et al., "Neural circuitry underlying the interaction between emotion and asthma symptom exacerbation," National Academy of Sciences, August, 2005.

86. Sternberg, E., "The Mind-Body Interaction in Disease," *Scientific American*, 1997.

87. Harrington, A., "Emotions and Disease," Natl. Library of Medicine Exhibit, History of Medicine Division, 1996.

88. Goleman, D., <u>Emotional Intelligence</u>, Bantam Books, 1996.

89. Davidson, J.R., Kabat-Zinn, J., "Alterations in Brain and Immune Function Produced by Mindfulness Meditation," *Psychosomatic Medicine*; 65: 564-570; 2003.

90. Flanders Dunbar, H., <u>Emotions and Bodily Changes: A Survey of Literature on Psychosomatic Interrelationships, 1910-1933</u>, New York, 1935.

91. Sontag, S., <u>Illness as Metaphor</u>, Picador, 1978.

Chapter 4

92. Ob cit, Pert, C.

93. Ob cit, Pert, C.

94. Harrington, A., "Emotions and Disease," Natl. Library of Medicine Exhibit, History of Medicine Division, 1996.

95. Schmeck, H., "By Training the Brain, Scientists Find Links to Immune System Defense," *The New York Times*, Jan. 1, 1985.

96. Pert, C., <u>Molecules of Emotion: The Science Behind Mind-Body Medicine</u>, Scribner, 1997.

97. Justice, B., <u>Who Gets Sick</u>, Peak Press, 2000.

98. "Stem cells could repair brain damage," *BBC News*, Tuesday, 21 January, 2003.

Chapter 5

99. Kandel, E., Ibid.

100. Ibid, Pert, C., <u>Molecules of Emotion: The Science Behind Mind-Body Medicine</u>.

101. Sternberg, E., *The Balance Within*, W.W. Freeman, 2001.

102. Damasio, A., <u>Descartes Error</u>, Penguin, 2005.

103. Wismer Fries, A., "Early experience in humans is associated with changes in neuropeptides critical for regulating social behavior," *Proceedings of the Natl. Academy of Sciences*; 102: 17237-17240; 2005.

104. Rudavsky, Shari, "Researcher Finds Brain Changes in Game Players," *The Indianapolis Star*, December 5, 2006.

105. Ibid, Damasio, A.

106. Pinker, S., <u>How the Mind Works</u>, W.W. Norton & Co.,1997.

107. Siegel, D., <u>The Developing Mind</u>, Guilford, 1999.

108. Zeki, S., "The Visual Image in Mind and Brain," <u>The Scientific American: Book of the Brain</u>, Lyons Press, 1999.

109. Crick, F. and Koch, C., "The Problem of Consciousness," *Scientific American*, 1997.

110. Goleman, D., <u>Social Intelligence: The New Science of Human Relationships</u>, Bantam, 2006.

111. Blakeslee, S., "Cells that Read Minds," *The New York Times*, January 10, 2006.

Chapter 6

112. Ibid, Seaward, B.

113. Green, E., <u>Beyond Biofeedback</u>, Delacorte Press, 1982.

114. McEwen, B., *Journal of Psychiatry & Neuroscience*, 30:315-318, 2005.

115. Cohen, S., "The Pittsburgh Common Cold Studies: Psychosocial predictors of susceptibility to respiratory infectious illness," *International Journal of Behavioral Medicine*, 12: 123-131; 2005.

116. Kiecolt-Glaser, J. K., et al., "Hostile marital interactions, pro-inflammatory cytokine production, and wound healing," *Arch Gen Psychiatry*, 62:1377-1384, 2005.

117. Gureje, O., et al., "Persistent Pain and Well-being: A World Health Organization Study in Primary Care," *Journal of American Medical Association*, 280(2): 147-51, 1998.

118. Baer, M., "Circadian Clock Genes May Provide Targets for New Cancer Drugs," American Association for Cancer Research, November 18, 2003.

119. "Heart Disease in Women," *Circulation*; 113: 463, January 31, 2006.

120. "How being black affects your blood pressure," Mayo Foundation for Medical Information and Research, April, 2005.

121. Hansson, GK, "Mechanisms of Disease: Inflammation, Atherosclerosis, and Coronary Artery Disease," *New England Journal of Medicine*, 352:1685-1695, Apr 21, 2005.

122. Sarno, J., <u>The Divided Mind</u>, Harper-Collins, 2006.
123. LeDoux, J., <u>The Emotional Brain</u>, Touchstone, 1996.
124. Goleman, D., <u>Emotional Intelligence</u>, Bantam Dell, 1995.
125. Kessler, R., *Archives of General Psychiatry*, 63:669-678; 2006.
126. Johnson, S., <u>Mind Wide Open</u>, Scribner, 2004.
127. Kandel, E., et al., <u>Principles of Neural Science</u>, McGraw-Hill, 2000.
128. Ibid, LeDoux, J.

Chapter 7
129. Houston, W., "The Doctor Himself as a Therapeutic Agent," *Annals of Internal Medicine*, 11: 1418; 1938.
130. Hróbjartsson A, et al, "Is the placebo powerless? An analysis of clinical trials comparing placebo with no treatment," *New England Journal of Medicine*;344:1594-602, 2001.
131. Benedetti F, et al, "Neurobiological mechanisms of the placebo effect," *Journal of Neuroscience*; 25:10390-402, 2005.
132. Barsky A.; et al., "Nonspecific Medication Side Effects and the Nocebo Phenomenon," *Journal of American Medical Association*; 287: 622 – 627; February 2002.
133. Kong J, et al, "Brain activity associated with expectancy-enhanced placebo analgesia as measured by functional magnetic resonance imaging," *Journal of Neuroscience*; 26:281-8; 2006.
134. Benson, H., "Mind/Body Interactions and Their Potential Clinical Applications," US Senate Appropriations Subcommittee on Labor/HHS & Education, September 22, 1998.
135. Wagner, T., et al., "Placebo-Induced Changes in fMRI in the Anticipation and Experience of Pain," *Science*; Vol. 303: 5661; February 20, 2004.
136. Zubieta JK et al, "Placebo effects mediated by endogenous opioid activity on mu-opiod receptors," *Journal of Neuroscience*, 25(34):7754–62; 2005.
137. Talbot, M., "The Placebo Prescription," *New York Times Magazine*, January 9, 2000.
138. Osler, W., <u>Principles and Practice of Medicine</u>, Pentland, 1892.
139. Ibid, Cousins, N.
140. Guarneri, M., <u>The Heart Speaks</u>, Touchstone Books, 2006.
141. Kirsch, I., *Prevention and Treatment*, 5: 23, July 15, 2002.
142. Ibid, Talbot.
143. Ob cit, Talbot.
144. Porter, R., <u>The Greatest Benefit to Mankind</u>, Norton Press, 1997.
145. Ob cit, Cousins, N.
146. Reid, B., "The Nocebo Effect: Placebo's Evil Twin," *The Washington Post*, April 30, 2002.
147. Ernst, F., et al., "Drug-Related Morbidity and Mortality: Updating the Cost-of-Illness Model," *Journal of the American Pharmaceutical Association*, Mar-Apr; 41(2):192-9; 2001.
148. Doskoch, P., "Happily Ever After," *Psychology Today*, 29: 32-34, 1996.
149. Ob cit, Cousins.

Chapter 8
150. Gureje, O., et al., "Persistent Pain and Well-being: A World Health Organization Study in Primary Care," *Journal of American Medical Association*, 280(2): 147-51, 1998.
151. "OxyContin Abuse and Diversion and Efforts to Address the Problem," US Government Accounting Office, GAO, 04-110, December 2003.
152. Kaufman, M. "Pitching Relief: A Physician with Firsthand Knowledge About Pain Advocates Opium-Based Drugs Despite Fears of Abuse," *Washington Post*, April 23, 2006.
153. Denizet-Lewis, B., "An Anti-Addiction Pill?" *The New York Times*, June 25, 2006.
154. Sarno, J., <u>The Divided Mind</u>, Harper-Collins, 2006.
155. "The History of the Relief of Pain & Suffering," The Louise M. Darling Biomedical Library, University of California, Los Angeles, 1998.
156. Ibid, Denizet-Lewis, B.
157. McGeary, D., "High Pain Ratings Predict Treatment Failure in Chronic Occupational Musculoskeletal Disorders," *The Journal of Bone and Joint Surgery (American)*; 88:317-325; 2006.
158. Mackey S., "Functional Imaging and the Neural Systems of Chronic Pain," *Neurosurgery Clinics of North America*, July 2004, Vol. 15, No. 3; 269-288.
159. Scholz J, Woolf, CJ, "Can we conquer pain?" *Nature Neuroscience*; 5: 1062-1067; 2002.
160. Ramachandran, V.S. and Blakeslee, S., <u>Phantoms in the Brain: Probing the Mysteries of the Human Mind</u>, William Morrow & Company, 1998.
161. Ramachandran, V.S, Altschuler, E. L. & Stone, L., et al.,"Can mirrors alleviate visual hemineglect?" *Medical Hypotheses*, vol. 52, no. 4, pp. 303-305; 1999.
162. "Most Americans older than 25 are overweight," CNN.com, March 5, 2002.

163. Vinik A., "Diabetic neuropathies," *Med Clin North Am.*; 88(4): 947-99; 2004.
164. Center for Disease Control and Prevention, Chronic Disease Prevention, US Dept. of Health and Human Services, 2005.
165. Green, GA, "*Understanding NSAIDS: from aspirin to COX-2*," *Clinical Cornerstone*; 3:50-59; 2001.
166. Berman, B., "Effectiveness of acupuncture as adjunctive therapy in osteoarthritis of the knee: a randomized, controlled trial," *Ann. of Internal Med.*; 141(12):901-10; 2004.
167. Vallfors B. Acute, "Subacute and Chronic Low Back Pain: Clinical Symptoms, Absenteeism and Working Environment," Scan J Rehab Med Suppl 1985; 11: 1-98.
168. The Merck Manual of Diagnosis and Therapy, Merck & Co. 2006.
169. Keogh, E., "Women feel pain more than men, research shows," *Medical News Today*, July 4, 2005.
170. Center for Research on Pain, The Hebrew University, Jerusalem.
171. Douglas, J. "Painkiller Patch Abuse Blamed for Deaths," *Washington Post*, June 15, 2006.
172. Kroenke K., "Studying symptoms: sampling and measurement issues," *Annals of Internal Medicine*, 134:844-53, 2001.
173. Ibid, Thernstrom, M., "My Pain, My Brain."
174. NIH Guide: "New Directions in Pain Research;" PA-98-102; 1998.

Chapter 9
175. Didion, J., The Year of Magical Thinking, Knopf, 2005.
176. Bajaj, V. "AN ENRON CHAPTER CLOSES: AN OBITUARY; Kenneth L. Lay, 64, Enron Founder and Symbol of Corporate Excess," *The New York Times*, July 5, 2006.
177. Simons, M., "Slobodan Milosevic, 64, Former Yugoslav Leader Accused of War Crimes, Dies," *The New York Times*, March 12, 2006.
178. Guarneri, M., The Heart Speaks, Touchstone, 2006.
179. Guimont, C., et al., "Chronic job strain may raise blood pressure," *American Journal of Public Health*, August 2006.
180. Reid, B., "Think Sick, Be Sick: The Nocebo Effect: Placebo's Evil Twin," *The Washington Post*, April 30, 2002.
181. Ibid, Guimont, C.
182. Nielsen, KM, "Danish singles have a twofold risk of acute coronary syndrome," *Journal of Epidemiology and Community Health*; 60:721-728; 2006.
183. Wansink, B., *Mindless Eating*, Bantam Books, 2006.
184. Lavelle, P. "Anger trigger to heart disease found?" *ABC Science Online*, 2003.
185. World Health Organization, "The World Health Report 2001: Mental Health: New Understanding, New Hope."
186. Hughes, J., *American Heart Journal*, May 2006.
187. Emery, C., et al., "Short-term effects of exercise and music on cognitive performance among participants in a cardiac rehabilitation program," *Heart & Lung*, 34: 4, July 2005.
188. Ibid, Guarneri, M.
189. Ibid, Guarneri, M.
190. Ornish, D., "Love Is Real Medicine," Newsweek, October 3, 2005.
191. Ibid, Guarneri, M.
192. Ibid, Ornish, D.

Chapter 10
193. Gershon, M., The Second Brain, HarperCollins, 1998.
194. Drossman DA et al, "AGA technical review on irritable bowel syndrome," *Gastroenterology*, 123: 2108–2131, 2002.

Chapter 11
195. Feingold, K., et al., "Glucocorticoid blockade reverses psychological stress-induced abnormalities in epidermal structure and function," *The American Physiological Society*, December 1, 2006.
196. Singer, N., "SKIN DEEP; If You Think It, It Will Clear," *The New York Times*, July 28, 2005.
197. Ibid, Singer.
198. Edelson, E., "Acne worsens at exam time," *HealthDay*, August 21, 2003.

Chapter 12
199. Hopkin, M., *Nature*; 440, 1096-1097, April 27, 2006.
200. Reid, D., The Complete Book of Chinese Health and Healing, Shambhala Publications, 1994.
201. Ibid, Reid, D.
202. Ob cit, Reid, D.

Chapter 13

203. Goleman, D., Mind-Body Medicine, Consumer Reports Books, 1993.
204. Epstein, M., Thoughts Without a Thinker, Harper Collins, 1995.
205. Ibid, p. 102.
206. Nyanatiloka, The Word of the Buddha, Buddhist Publication Society, 1971.
207. Ibid, Nyanatiloka.
208. Goleman, D., Destructive Emotions: How Can We Overcome Them? Bantam Books, 2000.
209. HH Dalai Lama, *Training the Mind: Verse 1*, 2006.

Chapter 14

210. Chopra, D., Perfect Health: A Complete Mind Body Guide, Three Rivers Press, 1991.
211. Blumer, R., The New Medicine, Middlemarch Films, 2006.
212. Chopra, D., Perfect Health, Three Rivers Press, 1991.

Chapter 15

213. Xue-Jun Song, et al., "Spinal manipulation reduces pain and hyperalgesia after lumbar intervertebral foramen inflammation in the rat," *Journal of Manipulative and Physiological Therapeutics*; 29(1):5-13; 2006; and Julita A., et al., "Spinal manipulative therapy reduces inflammatory cytokines but not substance P production in normal subjects," *Journal of Manipulative and Physiological Therapeutics*; 29(1):14-21; 2006.
214. Gudavalli R, et al., "A randomized clinical trial and subgroup analysis to compare flexion-distraction with active exercise for chronic low back pain," *European Spine Journal*, 2005.
215. Cox JM, Low Back Pain: Mechanism, Diagnosis, Treatment, 6th ed., Williams & Wilkins Publishers, 1999.
216. Murphy DR: et al, "A non-surgical approach to the management of lumbar stenosis: a prospective observational cohort study," *BMC Musculoskelet Disord*; 7:16; 2006.
217. Kadanka A,et al, "Approaches to spondylotic cervical myelopathy: conservative versus surgical results in a 3 year follow up study," *Spine*; 27(20); 2002.
218. Wolske A, Eisenberg D, et al, "Patterns and perceptions of care for treatment of back and neck pain," *Spine*; 28(3); 2003.
219. Dyer WW, There's a Spiritual Solution to Every Problem, Quill of Harper Collins Publishers, 2001.
220. Delport, J., et al, "104 patients over age 55 diagnosed with spinal stenosis response to epidural injection," *Archives of Physical Medicine and Rehabilitation*; 85(3); 2004.
221. Valet B., et al, "Epidural corticosteroid injections for sciatica: a randomized, double blind, controlled clinical trial," *Annals of the Rheumatic Diseases*; 62(7); 2003.
222. Atlas SJ., et al, "Long term outcomes of surgical and non surgical management of sciatica secondary to a lumbar disc herniation: 10 year results from the Maine Lumbar Spine Study," *Spine*; 30(8):927-35; 2005.
223. Fairbank J., et al, "Randomized controlled trial to compare surgical stabilization of the lumbar spine with an intensive rehabilitation programme for patients with chronic low back pain: The MRC spine stabilization trial," *British Medical Journal*; 330(7502):1233-39; 2005.
224. Kolata, G., "Surgery Need Is Questioned in Disc Injury," *The New York Times*, November 22, 2006.

Chapter 16

225. Saul, Stephen, "Study Links Ambien Use to Unconscious Food Forays," *The New York Times*, March 14, 2006.
226. "Can't Sleep? Science Is Seeking New Answers," CAM at the NIH, Volume XII, Number 3: Summer 2005.

Chapter 21

227. "Heavy Metal Makes Killer Mice, Teen Finds," *Washington Times*, July 29, 1997.

Chapter 22

228. Robinson, V., "Humor in nursing," In C. Carlson & B. Blackwell, (Eds.), *Behavioral concepts and nursing interventions*, Lippincott, 1978.

About the Authors

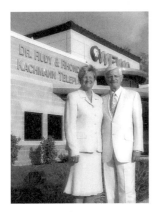

Rudy Kachmann, M.D., is the cofounder of the Kachmann Mind Body Institute in Fort Wayne, Indiana, and has practiced neurosurgery for over 40 years. Dr. Kachmann received his medical training from Georgetown University where he was Chief Resident of Neurosurgery, and Indiana University where he received his B.S. and M.D.

His research and lectures have been broadcast locally on PBS. His support of the arts, including sponsorship of the Unity Youth Choir and Kachmann Gallery have been featured many times in the local media, including radio and television broadcasts, newspapers, magazines, and community journals. He is the author of *Twenty Prescriptions for Living the Good Life* and producer of *Oh My Aching Back*.

Dr. Kachmann is on the Board of Directors of Day Break Children's Shelter and the Board of Trustees of Lutheran Hospital. He is the founder of the Kachmann Behavioral Foundation that funds community-based educational initiatives and member of the Tennis Hall of Fame. He has received several awards, including the Martin Luther King award for his support of community outreach. Dr. Kachmann is a long-time resident of Fort Wayne where he lives with his wife, Yorkshire terrier, and two Tonkinese cats.

Kim Kachmann-Geltz received a B.A. in humanities from Indiana University, and a M.A. in American Studies from Columbia University. Her writing career began as a legislative correspondent on Capitol Hill, and her knowledge of health care and medicine grew as the director of SpeakOutUSA, a non-profit that developed educational videos and produced health care reform hearings for bipartisan member of the U.S. Congress.

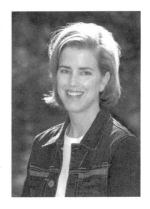

She joined America Online, Inc. as writer and editor of the "Welcome Screen" before becoming director of AOL International Content & Programming where she developed the company's first manual on editorial content standards and practices and taught the "best practices" to AOL's joint ventures in 11 different countries around the world.

Today she directs research and development for the Kachmann Mind Body Institute and is working with her father on their next book. She lives on Hilton Head Island with her husband, three young children, Yorkshire terrier, rabbit, and two Tonkinese cats.

The Kachmann Mind Body Institute will offer a variety of workshops, resources and educational opportunities on the campus of Lutheran Hospital in the fall of 2007. For information on the institute, please contact info@KachmannMindBody.com, or visit KachmannMindBody.com.

Kachmann Mind Body Institute
7950 W Jefferson Boulevard
Fort Wayne, IN 46804
USA